Praise for

BIRTH CONTROL

"The US has some of the worst maternal-health outcomes in the world, and the story of how birth went from a physiologic event to a medical event is an important one that has shaped the maternal- and infant-health trajectory of every birthing person in this country. *Birth Control* tells this critically important story with empathy, journalistic rigor, and vivid detail. A must-read for anyone who is considering, cares about, or came from a birth."

—Kimberly Seals Allers, author of *The Big Letdown*

"This fascinating, impassioned, and exhaustively researched book is a must-read for anyone who has ever been involved in childbirth—which is everyone. Allison Yarrow shines a light on misogyny in the American health care system and offers hope for what giving birth can look like when women, rather than profits, are centered."

—J. Courtney Sullivan, *New York Times*–bestselling author of *Friends and Strangers*

"Yarrow shines a light on a very dark truth: American obstetrics is failing women, too often putting profit over not only medical evidence but the interests and safety of pregnant, birthing, and new mothers. This book is a clarion call to physicians to do better by and for birthing people, and it's a reminder to those on the path to motherhood that they have the right to safe, respectful, and truly evidence-based care—which includes the ancient and the modern, the home and the hospital, and is best protected by midwives, doulas, and those who see birth as a natural, physiologic experience. It's time to relearn birth as a sacred event, not as the manufactured medical catastrophe waiting to happen that we've been indoctrinated to believe it is, and *Birth Control* points the way."

—Aviva Romm, MD, *New York Times*–bestselling author of *Hormone Intelligence*

Also by Allison Yarrow

*90s Bitch: Media, Culture, and the Failed Promise of
Gender Equality*

THE INSIDIOUS
POWER OF MEN
OVER MOTHERHOOD

BIRTH
CONTROL

ALLISON YARROW

SEAL PRESS

New York

Seal Press

Hachette Book Group

1290 Avenue of the Americas, New York, NY 10104

www.sealpress.com

Printed in the United States of America

First Edition: July 2023

Published by Seal Press, an imprint of Perseus Books, LLC, a subsidiary of Hachette Book Group, Inc. The Seal Press name and logo is a trademark of the Hachette Book Group.

The Hachette Speakers Bureau provides a wide range of authors for speaking events. To find out more, go to hachettespeakersbureau.com or email HachetteSpeakers@hbgusa.com.

Seal books may be purchased in bulk for business, educational, or promotional use. For information, please contact your local bookseller or Hachette Book Group Special Markets Department at special.markets@hbgusa.com.

The publisher is not responsible for websites (or their content) that are not owned by the publisher.

Print book interior design by Amy Quinn.

Library of Congress Cataloging-in-Publication Data
Names: Yarrow, Allison, author.
Title: Birth control: the insidious power of men over motherhood / Allison Yarrow.
Description: First edition. | New York, NY: Seal Press, [2023] | Includes bibliographical references and index.
Identifiers: LCCN 2023008853 | ISBN 9781541619319 (hardcover) | ISBN 9781541619326 (ebook)
Subjects: LCSH: Maternal health services—Moral and ethical aspects—United States—History. | Discrimination in medical care—United States—History. | Childbirth—United States—History. | Motherhood—United States—History.
Classification: LCC RG960 .Y37 2023 | DDC 362.198200973—dc23/eng/20230406
LC record available at https://lccn.loc.gov/2023008853

ISBNs: 9781541619319 (hardcover), 9781541619326 (ebook)

LSC-C

Printing 1, 2023

For those who have and those who will.

Some ideas are not really new but keep having to be affirmed from the ground up, over and over.

—Adrienne Rich, 1986

CONTENTS

AUTHOR'S NOTE

BIRTH CONTROL IS A WORK OF JOURNALISM AND NARRATIVE NON-fiction. It is not medical advice. Details of my life experience and the experiences of others are recounted faithfully and to the best of my ability. Some names and identifying characteristics have been changed to protect myself and others.

The people who give birth include some of the most vulnerable in our society. This book is for them all. I'll use the descriptors *woman* and *mother*, as most people who birth identify this way, and these are identities that widespread misogyny targets in specific ways that I document and describe here. Not using *woman* and *mother* could be considered its own form of misogyny.

I will also use the term *birthing people* to acknowledge and include those who give birth, but who don't identity as women or mothers. The necessary and important perspectives of gender nonbinary and trans birthing people inform my work. They are targets of hate and violence simply for being who they are, and this dynamic is magnified during pregnancy and childbirth. I hope this book speaks to their experiences and connects them to others who share those experiences.

At the same time, this book is not intended to fully capture the unique and difficult birth experiences of trans men. The challenges trans men and nonbinary people face during birth and the ways they are coerced and abused are both similar to and very different from what women endure. Their lives and interactions with the birth system are not my area of expertise or the focus of my research. There should be more books about and for them. They belong and deserve support during pregnancy, full stop.

The bottom line and the point I'm making is that, no matter who is laboring, the American childbirth experience is overwhelmingly and needlessly coercive, traumatic, tragic, harmful, and dangerous. The experience and outcomes for women and birthing people are worse as one ascends the scale of marginalization, as I will explore and explain throughout this book.

This book was written mostly during the time when *Roe v. Wade* still stood to protect our human right to abortion—that is, our ability to decide if, when, and how we become mothers and parents. *Roe* fell as I was readying the manuscript for publication. *Roe*'s collapse was many people's first exposure to the idea that institutions can control your body—that you are not in control of your own body. This revelation is a good introduction to pregnancy, childbirth, and motherhood in America. Ever wonder why childbirth is the most profitable hospital procedure? Or why it is a hospital procedure at all?

Killing *Roe* is an egregious example of reproductive rights disappearing, of our autonomy being usurped when many of us weren't looking. Our rights are being stripped from us during pregnancy and childbirth too. Sometimes it's because we're not paying attention. More often it is because structural patriarchy and white supremacy are foundational to perinatal care in this country. And yet, the depth of their reach is willfully concealed from us when we are vulnerable.

That's what this book is about. In ways large and small, our humanity, dignity, and well-being are violated during every aspect of pregnancy and childbirth, which I document here through extensive journalism, research, expert interviews, original survey data, and personal narrative. Since I have reported on and written about reproductive healthcare for more than a decade, I knew to expect some of this when I became pregnant for the first time—but that didn't stop sexism from shaping my childbirths too. Here's my best effort to ensure that it doesn't shape yours.

INTRODUCTION

REACH DOWN AND FEEL THE HEAD.

My midwife's words.

Just before: Do you want the mirror? Ben asks from the foot of the bed where he stands, holding its plastic handle aloft. It had arrived from Amazon the day before. I freed it from the box and plastic. Gripped the handle. Imagined my first glimpse of the baby inside me in that reflective square. How I would use that image as motivation.

Now, in this moment, I can't look in the mirror that I purchased for this purpose. I had wanted to desperately. But I can only shut my eyes. I need to go inside myself to allow labor to take over my body. Closing my eyes flings open that door. Inside to well up, ring out. Labor feels like a tide inside. Even the fluid within the uterus is saline, like the ocean.

I sense the internal wave drawing back and gathering speed and bulk. I feel the pressure of the water sucked from my body's interior walls, muscles, and arteries. Then the release, the crash, the push. Not an action I execute, but a sensation I withstand. If my mind can only get out of its way.

During my previous births, the power of my uterus contracting on its own had launched babies from my body. Now, my body pushes, but the waves pause instead of crash. I feel heat at the exit, a jerk like being grabbed by the collar. I snap backward to where the water doesn't hit the shore, dissolve into foam, or roll out again. What happened? I had expected that swell to send the baby out. A glint of doubt in my chest blocked the release.

Reach down and feel the head.

The words like a prophesy. A call. I elongate my arm, cover the opening with my palm. The head is mushy and warm. I can feel the damp tendrils of my baby's hair. That touch lights me from within. Feeling my baby makes my baby real. I gather up the strength not just to withstand the push again but to invite it. The water draws from everywhere in my body into a column. My neighbor later told me that she heard me wail through the wall, our headboards on either side of the same century-old brick and plaster, stuffed with newspaper clippings and horsehair. The wave thrashes forward, breaks to the surface. Foam and droplets shimmer in the air.

Ben and our midwife catch and place our infant, wet and wriggling, on my chest. She covers us in a towel, then stretches the cotton hat that I had laid out on the dresser over the tiny head. Aside from a brief, sharp cry, the baby is soundless. We bask in this majesty. We don't know or seek the sex; we just breathe into the peace of birth's aftermath.

The baby's skin is caked in vernix, a waxen white substance that they wash off in the hospital. Here in our bedroom no one touches it. I rub a little into the baby and into me like lotion. It regulates body temperature as the baby transitions from a liquid life to land, to breathing air. A few hours later it is gone, absorbed.

CHILDBIRTH IS THE MOST POWERFUL MOMENT OF A WOMAN'S LIFE, explains Sheila Kitzinger, the British birth advocate, activist, and author of more than two dozen books on the topic. She calls its force aquatic. "The power of birth is like the strength of water cascading down the hillside, the power of seas and tides, and of mountains moving. There is no way of ignoring it. You cannot fight it."

Birth as a natural force is woven through religion, art, literature, and the history of the world. It is "the Mount Everest of physical functions in any mammal," according to midwife Ina May Gaskin, whose *Guide to Childbirth* has become perinatal required reading. Gaskin describes the movement, the prolonged sensations, the shapeshifting of organs, the sheer exertion, as so vast that they are ineffable to the uninitiated. And yet, they are so fundamental and basic as to occur hundreds of thousands of times every day.

But I like the grounded aphorism best: A woman meets herself in childbirth.

It's what Cynthia Caillagh believed. She was one of the few remaining midwives still practicing in the style predating modern obstetrics, until her death in October 2022. She studied with a Cherokee midwife in Tennessee in the 1960s. In this tradition, birth invites self-knowledge while also "representing our greatest potential for what we can be as a species, if we let it teach us."

One could argue that we birth better than our mothers did. Today, half of American obstetricians are women, people who themselves could give or have given birth. Abundant information and education about birth exists, accessible to more people than ever before. We have greater accountability in medicine, safer and more effective drugs, and superior technology. More people take birth education classes, download apps, follow influencer accounts, read books, buy gear, and architect birth plans. We who birth today are better resourced and more knowledgeable. And yet, few of us experience labor and birth during which we are supported, listened to, and acknowledged as the experts in our bodies, in a place we feel comfortable, surrounded by affirmation and care so as to meet ourselves.

"Empowering" is not how most people describe childbirth. For most, birth is quite the opposite—disempowering, frightening, even threatening. Others control birth, not those doing it. Doctors, nurses, physicians' assistants, insurance companies, legislators, courts. Birth is dangerous, medicine is safe. That's the narrative, but it's far from the reality.

People are dying from childbirth in record numbers, a shocking occurrence given the advancements of our modern world. Only in recent decades have we begun to even count these deaths. When researchers first standardized data collection, they discovered that the maternal mortality rate in America more than doubled between 2000 and 2014. The rate rose again during the coronavirus pandemic. In 2019, 754 people died from childbirth in the US; in 2020, 861 did. In 2021, 1,205 died, which is a 40 percent increase in just one year, and the highest rate of death since 1965. While COVID may have exacerbated this tragedy, crisis-level outcomes in childbirth predate the pandemic by at least a century. Tragically, the majority of these deaths are preventable.

Unnecessary and unwanted surgical birth has likewise increased. Between 30 and 40 percent of American women describe their births as "traumatic." Trauma can be disguised by commonness; it also couldn't exist without disempowerment. The wholesale control of birth makes perverse sense when you consider who is being controlled: women of all colors, trans men, and nonbinary people—some of the most marginalized people in our society.

I'M OBSESSED WITH BIRTH STORIES, BUT FOR SO COMMON AN ACT, they're hard to come by, which is telling in and of itself. For the last decade, I've asked people about their pregnancies, childbirths, and transitions to motherhood. The first birth story I heard was from a friend who was too afraid to learn anything about birth. She complied with her doctor's orders during labor, but she tore badly while pushing, which she couldn't feel because she was anesthetized. I hurt for her, and her experience haunted me. But I was certain that it was unique to her. I couldn't have been more wrong.

In birth storytelling, the details variegate, but the takeaway is very often the same: birth didn't go as planned; it went haywire. Healthy people with normal pregnancies become patients with risks, diagnoses, near-death experiences, damage. They assume—or are told after the fact—that something was wrong with their body or their baby.

I wanted to confirm my strong feeling that something was deeply awry with the system of birth in our country. I wondered whether my suspicion was correct: Was the fact that I was hearing too many bad birth stories to count somehow a product of the people who gave birth? After all, in many cases, they reported to me that it was somehow their own fault.

Or did the blame lie elsewhere? At the feet of an overburdened hospital system pushing profits or the patriarchal and white supremacist structures that created and govern them? I wondered to what extent women and birthers believed these forces shaped their births and pregnancies. I wanted to explore the experiences of people who birth and become mothers today.

In 2019, I conducted a survey of birthing people, the results of which inform and appear throughout this book. The survey mostly contained quantitative, multiple-choice questions, but there were qualitative free-response prompts too. I shared it with my friends and colleagues, with my professional networks, and in online communities of parents and moms. I ensured that I reached groups underrepresented in pregnancy and birth research, namely, people who identify as Black, Latinx, Asian, and mixed race. I've been fortunate to collaborate with a team of researchers at the New School whose skills and insights were key to my understanding of what the data I collected could mean.

I never imagined that 1,307 people would take the survey. The number of participants, combined with the length and quality of the free responses, indicates that people hunger to share their birth experiences. Tellingly, I found that nearly 47 percent are rarely or never asked to tell their birth stories. Only 45 percent are asked to do so "occasionally." The majority of respondents were white women. The second-largest group surveyed identified as Black/African, followed by Hispanic/Latinx, and then Asian. Most survey respondents were married and identified as heterosexual, though a significant percentage identified as LGBTQ. The majority were between thirty and forty years old, gave birth in US cities, and graduated from college, and the group was relatively high earning. Income and education did not protect against birth that didn't go as expected or was described as traumatic. The longer a labor, the more likely respondents were to call it traumatic. The more time spent in the hospital, the worse their experience. Just being in the place where we're supposed to receive birth care is doing harm.

IN OUR SOCIETY, WE BUY EXPECTING MOTHERS BABY GIFTS. WE NOtice, comment on, and touch their changing bodies. We mostly ignore and fail to support their shifting selves. Baby arrives, and she's all we see. As if a literal stork dropped her off. The journey of the soul and body that gave birth aren't discussed. Most often, they're erased. No wonder more than 70 percent of those I surveyed believed that media depictions of pregnancy did not represent their experiences. Pregnancy turns our bodies into a new kind of public commodity and a receptacle for others' ideas about who we are. About 79 percent of people I surveyed said people touched or commented on their bodies while they were pregnant. Almost everyone.

Women enter pregnancy brimming with all they have learned from books, films, the internet, and experts. We bring into the labor ward the stories we've heard, coveted, or wished away. My greatest fear was surgical birth or tearing. I expended so much energy during my first pregnancy praying to avoid those things. Many of us experience birth as disappointment, manipulation, and (whether or not we use this word) abuse. Sometimes we feel this as it's happening; other times it goes unchecked, and we may need years to see it, if we ever do. We quietly blame a doctor who withheld support, a grouchy nurse, a problem with our body or baby that we internalize. Then we chastise ourselves for not having predicted or fixed it. We excuse bad judgments, unnecessary medicine we are "consented to," horrendous bedside manner, or lies that masquerade as care. And we are gaslit into believing all of this is lifesaving—for our baby, for ourselves.

We slough off that birth attendants refused to do what we asked or failed to ask us before doing things to our bodies. We turn the blame inward when elements of our births don't go to plan. If only we hadn't hoped for that natural birth so hard. Stupid to enter an orchard wishing for magic fruit. Or perhaps we should have learned more about C-sections in birth class—we could have avoided surgery or prepared for it. We vow not to plan so hard next time, not to get our hopes up, lest we be disappointed and feel blamed again. We accept the mantra that birth is unpredictable and that we're lucky, blessed, to leave with our lives intact and babies pulsing in our arms.

We don't live in birth long enough to see it for what it really is: a system built in tandem with a profession founded on fear of the generative power of the birthing body. Obstetrics is a specialty constructed in the belief that Black pregnant bodies tolerate more pain and are predisposed to disease, while white pregnant bodies' frailty requires expert control—medical arts, tools, drugs. The profession is highly skilled while simultaneously hamstrung by hospital systems for which maternity services turn the heftiest profit. Every birth is a manufactured healthcare crisis only doctors with rigid protocols in multi-million-dollar hospitals can solve. It is a system that has evolved to control women for money.

"It's amazing how profitable being bad at childbirth can be," Kavita Patel, a physician and former hospital executive who negotiated service prices with insurance companies for the federal government, told me. Hospitals are fundamentally terrible places for childbirth to occur. They are crammed with stress, sickness, cacophony, narcissism, toxic workplace dynamics, and harshness, from aesthetics to administration. Birthers are the only people seeking assistance at hospitals who aren't sick or injured. Patel likened the care to an assembly line: the more bodies churning through, the more money for the medical-industrial complex.

Hospitals are where about 98 percent of American childbirth occurs. We go to them for many reasons—among them, culture and convention, the law, and ignorance. We flee the safety and security of our homes and the people we love and trust most and yield our bodies to facilities that exist to stave off death and treat disease. We easily accept the idea that they are safe places to birth because their function is preservation.

But we are in female bodies, Black bodies, trans bodies, and our protection is not guaranteed. In the hospital, our well-being and sometimes our lives are needlessly put at risk. A bevy of technologies, policies, drugs, practitioners, and administrators control us. They tell us that we're too fast, too slow, too early, too late, too loud, too quiet, too much, not enough. These are familiar criticisms because, as women and birthing people, we hear them throughout our lives in other contexts. We come to know these condemnations like lovers. They first enter our thoughts and self-talk; then they worm into us, becoming not external modifiers but facts.

The truth is that no matter how much we learn about birth before having a baby, control is wrested from us with a sinister precision when birth day comes. We are told explicitly and implicitly that we are not experts in our own bodies, that strangers know best, that to be kept safe amid a tsunami of danger, we must submit to nameless faces who command with degrees, acronyms, mandatory procedures, protocols, monitoring, and a parade of fears. Physiological birth becomes not about nature, selfhood, or exaltation but about survival. And if you survive, well, even brutal means justify the end.

After hearing countless stories of coerced and controlled birth on repeat, I wasn't surprised to uncover them in my data. Survey participants who birthed with a male obstetrician were, statistically, significantly more likely to receive care they didn't want, consent to, or understand. They felt blamed or judged when labor or delivery didn't go as planned and as though their provider didn't take their pain or discomfort seriously. A quarter of women said that during labor, their providers appeared more concerned with the baby's safety than the mother's. All of these experiences—unwanted care, ignored pain, feeling blamed or judged, and more concern for babies than moms— were also present for those who delivered with a female obstetrician. The survey found a strong, statistical relationship between reporting birth trauma and feeling blamed or judged. None of these experiences were significantly connected to delivering with a midwife.

These findings sadly confirm that, as we birth, we are cut off from the full joy, wonder, and power of what birth is and should be, manipulated by a system that dominates by wielding fear. When a doctor tells us our baby is at risk, does a procedure to eliminate said risk, and then celebrates a healthy baby (thanks to *their* intervention), what could we possibly have to complain about? Then we are rushed out the door. We soldier on after birth. We take care of our kids and our families and don't revisit what feels too awful to sit with. Who has the time? We call it past and slam the door as we walk forward. We do it to survive.

Birth stories are powerful. They "teach us of possibilities that might not occur to us without them," mused midwife Ina May Gaskin. That's why, in addition to presenting extensive reporting, survey work, and interviews with experts and birthing people, this book is about how a system that usurps birthers' power shaped my own pregnancies and births. I'm reporting this, and I have lived it. I gave birth twice in the same Brooklyn hospital—first with a female nurse-midwife, then with a male obstetrician. My third birth was a planned home birth with a female midwife. In the pages that follow, I share the intricacies of my birth stories: how providers coerced me, how I triumphed, and how I gaslit myself during and after my hospital births. In Chapter 11, I share the intimacy of my home birth experience to demystify a stigmatized practice that more people should investigate and, I think, choose. Pandemic curiosity about home birth, catalogued in a raft of perturbed media reports, actually inspired much more of it. The rate spiked 22 percent from 2019 to 2020, the sharpest rise in the practice in about thirty years. Still, just over 1 percent of all births occur outside a hospital setting today.

MATERNAL MORTALITY HASN'T INCREASED BECAUSE PREGNANCY and birth in America are inherently and commonly deadly. The deepseated fear of death, pain, and injury in birth are exploited to enact routine medical procedures without consent, as I explore in Chapters 2 and 3. Mothers most often suffer and die from the overuse of controlling medicine, not when it is withheld.

There are many known contributing factors to our present maternal mortality scourge. The increased C-section rate drives poor outcomes, as I report in Chapter 6. About a third of births are surgical, which is at least double what's necessary. Short postpartum hospital stays, which contracted further during the pandemic, don't help: in 2020, some 73 percent of hospitals sent mothers and infants home less than forty-eight hours after birth. Postpartum hemorrhage is a leading cause of maternal death, and too often birthers are out the door before it occurs.

Serena Williams, one of the most famous athletes in the world, nearly died of postpartum hemorrhage. She believes that this was in no small part because she is Black. Black women are three to four times more likely to die from childbirth than white women. Racism and implicit bias in healthcare and society have produced poorer care. Historically, Black women were believed to be heartier and more pain tolerant in early medicine and obstetrics, outlandishly bigoted and discredited theories that, as I'll explain in Chapter 1, infiltrate care today.

The environment and the cultural ideas that surround women directly affect whether they survive birth. One out of every five women of reproductive age in southern states lives in a county with a high risk of death from childbirth and other serious problems, including postpartum hemorrhage, preeclampsia, and preterm birth. Underlying disease, homelessness, and food insecurity negatively impact birth. Nonwhite women are more likely to live in places that threaten their births. Researchers at a health-data nonprofit wrote about these trends in the *New York Times* in 2021, calling them "shameful" and imploring the United States to probe the quality of birth care along with "the entire environment around [the mother]—from her access to health care to the availability of food in her community." We are just beginning to acknowledge that bad birth outcomes and deaths result not only from poor birth care but also from a world that is toxic to women, most of all women of color.

Women are subject to abuse and even assault during birth, but rarely do they receive justice or even any acknowledgment that they suffered. Instead, they hear they were rescued by procedures, as I explain in Chapter 5, or their bodies were flawed from the start (that's Chapter 4). Birth trauma survivors told researcher Cheryl Beck they felt "raped on the table with everyone watching and no one to help." Beck says she has heard a version of that statement countless times. I document a grotesque case of such abuse in Chapter 7 and argue that being "consented to" exams or procedures—terminology to describe when women are instructed to have, or coerced into having, certain medical care—must end.

It's no surprise that controlled birth leads to mental health problems, like depression, anxiety, and posttraumatic stress disorder. As I explore in Chapter 10, these consequences impact not just individuals but generations of families. The dearth of support for postpartum conditions that afflict new moms, which I cover in Chapter 8, fuels mental health challenges, as does a society that sings "Breast Is Best" while actively thwarting breastfeeding initiation and continuation (Chapter 9).

Because the experience of birth is personal, we forget that it is also political. We know that countless women struggle during pregnancy, childbirth, and new motherhood, but we aren't discussing these problems through the lens of systemic sexism, racism, and inequality. In fact, our society doesn't view the problems of mothers and motherhood as real problems at all. We attribute these struggles to individual women who then blame themselves for systemic shortcomings. We must first recognize and believe that misogyny, sexism, and racism shape birth before we can upend them.

"Mom problems" are patronized as soft, unserious, and unworthy of real consideration, let alone solutions. Paid leave was axed when it weighed down the Infrastructure Investment and Jobs Act of 2021. Politicians in both parties failed to see it as relevant to building the country. Mothers' prostrations of pain and childcare crises unfold in what has become a genre of news article, but no matter how many stories stack up, nothing is done. We're left screaming in the dark on empty ball fields, like mothers in Massachusetts and New York famously did during the pandemic.

Our struggles, anger, and pain are real, and they are impeding the progress of our country and our species. We should interrogate the science, healthcare, policy, economics, marketing, systems, language, and cultural mores that promote a patriarchal, white status quo in childbirth and maternal healthcare. Poet Adrienne Rich reminds us that "alienated childbirth, botched illegal abortions, needless

cesareans, involuntary sterilizations, individual encounters with arro-
gant and cavalier physicians were never mere anecdotes, but testimony
through which the neglect and abuse of women by the healthcare system could be substantiated." Our stories and knowledge should inspire new institutions and systems to serve our needs.

The systemic patriarchy and white supremacy foundational to modern perinatal healthcare must be first understood and then disman-
tled to save lives, improve birth for all, strengthen our families, and
better our society. Reproduction and birth are about power—who has
it and who doesn't. The people doing the procreating don't. Birth must
return to our control. Our lives depend on it.

CHAPTER 1
WELCOME TO PREGNANCY

Sloane, Valerie, and Olivia are talking to me about the periods they will one day have. They are ten-year-olds in the final days of fifth grade before summer 2019. I tell them that in my reporting, I'm finding that grown women don't know much about their menstrual cycles, or ovulatory cycles, as researchers call them. I am seated across from them in a low chair. From over the top of my very pregnant stomach, I ask what they are learning about menstruation, ovulation, and sex, about bodies that do these things?

"We're really not," Valerie says, elbow deep in a carton of Goldfish. Crunching sounds will punctuate our three-hour conversation, during the course of which the girls will sit on the couch, on the ground, talk over each other, fetch things from the kitchen, and scroll their phones. When they identify with what another of them is saying, they murmur, "Same."

Recently, they withstood a two-day puberty lecture from a guest facilitator brought in by their public elementary school in Brooklyn. Boys and girls were not separated—they heard everything together, at the same time.

"All they told us about it was that it was a part of puberty where you got blood in your private parts and then you would have to wear pads and tampons or whatever to help, so the blood can't get out," Sloane says, swinging on Olivia's crutches. A basketball injury put Olivia in a black cast that stretches from her ankle to her thigh.

"They say that it kind of makes you freak out," Valerie adds, tugging her green bucket hat. A friend got her period and told Valerie the biggest burden was petitioning teachers to use the bathroom during school. The girls' foremost concern is the difficulty and shame of period logistics. Not helpful, they add, is the lack of supplies readily available at school. They're not in the bathroom; you have to go to the nurse.

If Valerie first bleeds at school, she plans to wad up toilet paper to make a temporary pad. If she's at home, she'll fetch one from beneath the sink. Sloane and Valerie will tell their moms immediately. Olivia will wait to assess her mom's mood.

Sentimentality or celebration would be unwelcome. Nobody wants to hear how they're "becoming a woman" or "growing up so fast"—that would be "awkward!" They won't discuss getting a period with their dads or siblings. In fact, our conversation halts when Sloane's slightly older brother arrives. When reminded that his mother has barred him from the room, he screeches conspicuously, then tries to spy from the top of the stairs.

I witness Sloane, Valerie, and Olivia make a pact to tell each other when they get their periods. They are fearful of telling people who can't keep secrets and of boys finding out. "I don't want them to look at me differently. Like I'm older or something," Valerie says.

When I ask whether the school talk might have gone better without boys in the room, they all agree that it would have. "It was harder to focus because a lot of the boys were kind of creeped out, because none of them really knew what a period was," Valerie says.

Olivia was distracted by a boy next to her. "And he was like, 'It's so embarrassing,' and I'm like, "'Can you stop? I'm trying to listen,'" she says.

"I'd be more comfortable with just girls because I feel like I can ask questions that, like, wouldn't make the boys start laughing," Valerie says.

The facilitator showed charts of reproductive organs. Sloane said the boys' chart was simple, as it consisted of "just, like, sperm, and penis, and a butt," but the girls' chart was confusing—"because so many parts."

They talked a lot about what happened to boys.

"Like when they have an ah-raction? Er-ection?" Sloane isn't sure of the pronunciation. The others try.

"Erie?" asks Olivia.

"Ir-ocktion?" asks Valerie. They look at me to settle it, which I do.

"Erection!" they say in unison.

"But no, there was something else too," Valerie says.

"Ejaculation?" I ask.

"Yeah, ejaculation," they say.

"You, like, touch the outline," Olivia explains to me.

"The ejaculation is when you . . ." Sloane starts. Valerie finishes her sentence. "When you rub your penis," she says. Olivia looks confused.

"Which one's the one where you . . ." Sloane begins again.

"That's masturbation," Valerie interrupts. So many same-suffixed words.

"Yeah, they're all *tion*," Sloane says. "Is that where the sperm comes out or where the penis is stiff?" Olivia has a different take. "Masturbation is kind of like the girl's period. You rub yourself and stuff comes out of you."

Valerie has another idea. "No, I think masturbation is more like when you want to reproduce but, like, it just feels good."

"Like a wet dream," Sloane says.

"We talked a lot about wet dreams," Olivia says.

Parsing the three *tions*—erection, ejaculation, and masturbation—revealed how the talk had preoccupied the girls with what happens to bodies with penises. The simple anatomy chart, followed by detailed explanations of wet dreams and impending orgasms, signaled that boys' puberty was something exciting to covet. The more complex female anatomy diagram, coupled with discussions of blood, menstrual products, mood swings, and pain, telegraphed that girls should expect discomfort and inconvenience.

The linchpin of puberty, they were taught, was that everyone will "have stuff that comes out." Sperm for boys, blood for girls. But while one is wanted and feels good, the other is unpredictable, uncontrollable, and requires hiding and cleaning. They imagined that intercourse was best avoided because it was painful and would lead to unwanted pregnancy. The only birth control discussed was condoms, which the girls labeled as "for boys." They didn't learn about what kind of contraception was "for girls." They also didn't discuss that pregnancy can only occur a few days each month; Valerie was surprised to learn this from Olivia and Sloane, who had heard it from their moms.

"I feel like masturbation is more about when you really want to have sex but not when you want to have babies," Valerie muses.

"Masturbation is when you touch yourself," Sloane says.

"Yeah. This stuff comes out, kind of like when this stuff comes out of your vagina," Olivia says.

"They talked about how when you masturbate, how when a boy masturbates, they also have an ejaculation," Sloane says.

"The boys can make themselves do it. They want to. But girls can't," Valerie says.

"We can't *make* ourselves have our periods," Olivia tells her, going for the Goldfish.

"No, masturbation," Valerie corrects.

"We can't make ourselves masturbate either," Olivia says, chewing.

"If we masturbate, we don't get our periods," Sloane says, certain.

Olivia turns to me. "Yeah, it made the boys feel better when they masturbated. More comfortable," she says.

"They didn't talk about that for girls," Valerie says.

Sloane bolts up. "Girls masturbating!?" she shouts. "What?"

Tellingly, there was no mention of the possibility of female pleasure. As if seeking distraction from this injustice, Sloane, Valerie, and Olivia spontaneously launch into a synchronized dance, miming someone's phone open to TikTok.

Their lesson lacked in other ways, starting with the facilitator's tendency to downplay the fifth graders' real concerns. "She was all, like, 'It's going to be fine, you have nothing to worry about,' when, like, we do, because we don't *want* to get our periods," Valerie says. "And the boys, like, I'm sure they have things that they worry about too. She made everything seem better than it was. She was avoiding the reality."

I'm likely saying what's obvious here, but these ten-year-olds were exceptionally smart. Rather than accept an incomplete picture, they preferred to hear about what periods are actually like—even just one person's experience. I am certain that they could hold the truth, or at least sit with their questions, as well as any adult. I could have told them what it was like for me, but I didn't. It wasn't appropriate. Or maybe I told myself that to avoid sharing and feeling attendant shame.

Meeting these girls, I had hoped to hear that sex education was different now than it had been when I was a kid. That it was more open and thoughtful, including not only anatomy but feelings, and that it invited participants to question and challenge what they were told. But here was history repeating itself. It felt like a fist to my chest.

Periods, to these ten-year-olds, were things of dread. Not only because they were poorly explained but because they differentiated you at a time when sameness carries reward. These girls believed—like I had, like plenty of girls do now—that identity is fixed and that beginning to ovulate is no milestone, not a tell about health, but a chore. A burden. They were told that this information about their bodies, about them, was biological, settled, accepted. That it couldn't be up for interpretation or questioning. That it couldn't be outright wrong.

"Sexism socially constructs female bodies as fundamentally flawed and in need of constant improvement, through engagement with consumer culture," according to Chris Bobel, a professor of gender studies at the University of Massachusetts and author of multiple books on menstruation, which she says is usually framed as "little more than a nuisance that must be cleaned up."

Menstruation's lack of appeal allows it to be easily hijacked. We are taught that periods are disposable. And sure enough, hundreds of millions of people worldwide, during the course of their fertile lives, won't actually have one. I didn't have one for the better part of thirteen years.

When I went to college, I got the pill because it symbolized freedom, adulthood, and the power to fuck with abandon. I wasn't doing that, but genuine desire coupled with an overdose of patriarchal conditioning had me wanting to believe that I could.

I drove to the campus health center rehearsing a pitch because I was terrified that the doctor would say no. I braced for my first pelvic exam, sure he would do one to properly assess whether I deserved and could safely take birth control. The doctor was tall, with tufts of hair cresting over his ears. He removed a pad from his coat pocket, scribbled, tore, and handed the top sheet to me. No pelvic exam or conversation. He didn't even tell me the drug's name, which I learned when a pharmacist filled the prescription. Orthotrycyclen came in a round case, a trinket, soothingly pink. I skimmed the instructions and ate a tablet twice the size of the mole on my cheek.

In the following months, my pants refused to zip. I gained the most weight at once that I ever had in my life, even though I walked everywhere, exercised regularly, and played soccer. I never suspected birth control was a culprit. I blamed myself—my drinking, my food choices. Sex was intermittently pleasurable (too often I was centering the wrong person), and that continued. My skin was clear, and my periods, or what I thought of as periods, were light and easy, only a pair of days each month. Sometimes I would skip the week of sugar pills that the packs contain to reassure you that you're not pregnant with a fake bleed. I'd head straight into another pack, just so I didn't have to bleed at all. Like, if I was going on vacation or sleeping with someone. My breasts grew so huge that I switched to bras without padding. My skin was as clear and soft as a baby's arm.

Then a friend told me about a birth control pill that contained less estrogen. She said that it didn't make you fat. I trucked back to the campus health center. Again, no exam, questions, or conversation. I started on Aviane the same day. My skin stayed clear, my breasts remained grapefruits on pesticide, and the weight melted off.

Informed consent is a central pillar of modern medicine. When professionals offer drugs or treatments, we should only choose them if we want them and after their risks and benefits are explained. My experience receiving the pill without explanation, conversation, or question mirrors that of most people who take hormonal birth control, according to Lisa Hendrickson-Jack, a fertility educator and author of *The Fifth Vital Sign*, a book on ovulatory cycles.

It became a nothingburger, the birth control. I forgot I was on it, never mentioning it on medical forms that inquired about prescription drugs. Even as more than a decade passed, I would never have a real conversation about it with a doctor. I graduated, moved to New York City. I got a job, a bed, an apartment, and a husband, in that order. Years later, I stopped taking pills to have kids.

Planned Parenthood's website touts, "The pill makes your period a breeze." Actually, it makes your period disappear by suppressing your ovulatory cycle. Doctors hardly ever discuss ovulatory suppression with their patients. Nor do we understand the impact of long-term hormonal birth control use on fertility, pregnancy, and birth. I reached my thirties without understanding how my reproductive system functions—that I could only get pregnant a few days each month—and what birth control actually does. About 27 percent of my survey respondents—some 350 people—agreed that they didn't know how menstrual cycles and ovulation worked before attempting pregnancy.

Hormonal birth control has improved and even saved lives by allowing people to plan their families. It also prevents pregnancy by crippling the reproductive system, which does far more for bodies than incubate babies. Hormonal birth control rewires the body and the mind, no matter the form. Pills and long-acting reversible contraception like intrauterine devices, patches, and shots all block production of vital hormones—estradiol and progesterone most of all—and replace them with counterfeits. The fake hormones mess with the endocrine system, the many glands that are responsible for metabolism, growth, hormone secretion, sleep, and mood, among other things. The changes are not small. They can cause harm—depression, diminished libido and orgasm, painful sex, weight gain, fatigue, brain fog—things women have speculated and secretly whispered about, and been told they were hallucinating, for years.

"Women aren't taught about their fertility or their menstrual cycle," fertility educator Hendrickson-Jack told me. "We're taught we can throw away our menstruation. We're told that unless you're trying to get pregnant, it doesn't matter." It's one thing to not understand ovulation before getting a period for the first time—the situation Sloane, Valerie, and Olivia were in. It's an entirely different thing to not understand it while pursuing pregnancy.

The many women's health experts I spoke to affirm that it does matter—that the menstrual cycle is the fifth vital sign, equal in importance to your blood pressure, heart rate, temperature, and respiratory rate. Monitoring your menstrual cycle provides information about the state of your body and health. However, most people only become interested in their cycles when trying to conceive, like I did, without realizing they haven't been having a cycle at all.

CONCEPTION AND PREGNANCY PROVIDE AN EARLY WINDOW INTO how American society so spectacularly bungles the entire birth process. The first thing you learn after confirming a pregnancy is your "due date." You don't need a medical professional to ascertain it—internet due date calculators help you find it yourself. You simply enter the first day of your last menstrual period, and voilà. Since most care providers won't see a pregnant woman until she's around eight weeks along, calculating a major data point can provide a bit of comfort and make a pregnancy feel real before the physicality of it takes hold.

A due date can seem like the only fixed point during a maelstrom of change. We pregnant folks have come to cling to it like a life preserver. It can become the entire anchor of a pregnancy, not only for mom-to-be but for her community—obsessed and thought about for nine long months. We clear our calendars, alert the neighbors, and call upon our people for the day that, nature and medicine tell us, our baby will finally be earthside.

But due dates are almost always wrong. Only 5 percent of pregnant people give birth on their actual due date. That means 95 percent, the overwhelming majority, don't. I never did: my first was born the day after her due date, my second four days after it, and my third six days early. I was born two days late, my husband two weeks early. You likely weren't born on your mother's due date; nor will you probably give birth to your baby on theirs. Societally, we've accepted due dates as hard stops—on or before which we should expect baby to emerge. But if they're so often misleading and inaccurate, why do we even use them?

Men created due dates. In the mid-1700s, a professor of medicine and botany named Hermann Boerhaave postulated when conception occurred. Boerhaave said that women were "impregnated after the end of their period" and stated that out of one hundred births, "ninety-nine came about in the ninth month after the last menstruation by counting one week after the last period and by reckoning the nine months of gestation from that time."

Franz Carl Naegele, a professor of obstetrics at the University of Heidelberg, framed the conception theory we use today in the early 1800s, which he built on biblical scholarship and Boerhaave's assumption. "The usual calculation of the duration of pregnancy, namely, starting from the last menstruation is correct in most instances," Naegele wrote. However, like Boerhaave, Naegele is imprecise. He does not specify which day of a person's period we should count from. Not knowing whether to choose the first day or the last, nineteenth-century doctors did both. I read that British doctors once advocated adding five days to the first day of a woman's period, and Irish practitioners added seven days, like American ones, but to the last day of the period rather than the first. These three methods would render different due dates, meaning the same woman would have a different due date, depending on whether she delivered in England, Ireland, or America.

By the twentieth century, Naegele's framework appeared in American obstetric and gynecological texts. These texts credited Naegele's rule with being the most precise due date calculation, though they inexplicably determined that adding seven days to the *first* day of the last menstrual period and then nine months was the correct calculation. That's where the forty-week, or 280-day, pregnancy comes from.

Naegele's guideline predates modern medicine and is derived not so much from science as from observation and assumption, and modern criticisms of it abound. One claims his rule rests "on the common belief that human gestation was ten menstrual cycles in duration, and not on empirical data," while another says it isn't "based on any current evidence, and may not have even been intended by Naegele." And yet, today, American doctors use the first day of the last menstrual period, then add 280 days to it, to estimate a due date. Naegele's two-century-old strategy underpins due date calculators populating today's internet.

Naegele's method assumes that all women menstruate identically— that we all have perfect twenty-eight-day menstrual cycles, dutifully dropping eggs in unison on day fourteen. But synchronized ovulation is not reality. Factors as basic as stress, diet, travel, illness, and irregular bedtimes can alter cycles. Mine changes noticeably when I have a cold. If a woman's cycle is longer than twenty-eight days, Naegele's rule likely underestimates her due date. If her cycle is shorter, the rule overestimates it.

We often don't know enough about our own menstrual cycles to combat this pseudoscience. We learn to manage periods, not to understand the full, necessary ovulatory activities of our bodies. For many, a monthly underwear stain comes as a surprise. Only about half of women accurately recall when the first day of their last menstrual period was. But there's no estimating a due date on your own without this information. Plenty of pregnant people, then, likely guess.

To further complicate matters, even those who are certain of the first day of their last menstrual period may be wrong, thanks to the omnipresence of hormonal birth control. Since hormonal birth control puts a kibosh on the natural menstrual cycle and produces a fake bleed rather than a real period, women who become pregnant in the cycle or cycles immediately after quitting the pill may not know the first day of their last menstrual periods. It may not be knowable at all. It's not clear how many birthing people this affects, but 46 percent of my survey respondents said they stopped taking hormonal birth control to get pregnant.

Modern science and new measurement tools have revealed more flaws in Naegele's method. According to a 1990 study led by Robert Mittendorf from the Harvard School of Public Health, first-time mothers delivered eight days later than Naegele's rule predicted, and experienced mothers did so three days later. In 2001, Gordon Smith, a professor of obstetrics and gynecology at the University of Cambridge, studied 1,514 pregnant women to establish a normal duration of human pregnancy. His work, published in the journal *Human Reproduction*, provided a more nuanced understanding of gestation length. Like the Harvard study, Smith used the women's menstrual histories to date their pregnancies but then confirmed the dates with first-trimester ultrasounds to pinpoint exact gestational age, a higher measurement standard than the previous study had used. He too found that a forty-week gestation period was wrong—both for first-time mothers and for mothers giving birth again. In new moms, pregnancy lasted five days longer than Naegele assumed. In moms who had given birth before, it was three days longer. Using ultrasound to date a pregnancy, if done at the right time (more about that below), can produce more accurate pregnancy dating than last menstrual period dates alone.

In 2013, researchers published the Early Pregnancy Study, further identifying the exact dates of ovulation, conception, and implantation in 125 women by measuring their hormones throughout their cycles, getting the most precise readings possible. Pregnant people who use in vitro fertilization have the most accurate due date estimates—they know the exact day of conception, allowing the closest possible assessment of their due date. What the Early Pregnancy Study revealed was pretty shocking: normal pregnancy length in healthy people can vary up to thirty-seven days, or more than five weeks.

These three studies helped show that Naegele's due date estimates had been homogenizing both ovulation in women and the speed at which embryos implant and babies develop in utero. Embryos implant at different speeds. Those slower to implant also took longer to grow. All kinds of factors, like the length of the embryo's journey, the environment in a pregnant person's body, and genetics, can impact a baby's growth timeline. According to the Early Pregnancy Study, the first to measure pregnancy based on exact dates, birth within the thirty-seven-day window is in the normal range. Once again, Naegele's theory that all women menstruate, ovulate, and grow babies the same way was refuted. As the researchers put it, "Human gestation length varies considerably even when measured exactly."

DUE DATES AREN'T A TRIVIALITY OF PREGNANCY. ACCORDING TO the American College of Obstetricians and Gynecologists (ACOG), the professional organization of doctors who deliver babies, due date accuracy is an important public health concern. "This information is vital for timing of appropriate obstetric care; scheduling and interpretation of certain antepartum tests; determining the appropriateness of fetal growth; and designing interventions to prevent preterm births, postterm births, and related morbidities," the group wrote. Incorrect due dates can threaten safe and healthy birth.

Joshua Copel is vice chair of obstetrics, gynecology and reproductive sciences at Yale. I wanted to talk to him because he is an expert in first-trimester scans and also because he coauthored an ACOG and Society for Maternal-Fetal Medicine committee opinion on the importance of accurate due date estimation. He agrees that the term *due date* "can be misleading."

"We can cause harm by acting if we don't have to act," he told me. He elaborated that the harm could come on both sides of a miscalculated due date. On the one hand, premature birth is a concern. The birth team needs to know if a birth is happening earlier than it should be to reduce the risk of prematurity. Or a doctor, thinking a baby is late when they are not, might force them to be born too soon.

Copel gave a hypothetical example: "If we got her due date wrong and she goes into labor on August 5, but her due date was actually July 15 there are risks related to being post-term. And since we do some things electively in obstetrics, for example someone's had three prior caesareans, she's going to have another caesarean. We wouldn't want to do that before she hits thirty-nine weeks and zero days." Babies born before their time can face health complications, particularly respiratory ones, because their development was cut short. Trying to remove a baby too soon can compromise lung development.

The most common result of the widespread use of Naegele's rule is that doctors assume babies are ready to be born when they are not. One of the risks involves the practice of artificially inducing labor through the use of medications or methods that prompt uterine contractions to begin. Induction for medical reasons, like a pregnancy complication, is one thing. Induction based on due date estimates is quite another. While some medical professionals certainly believe and will try to convince women that inducing at thirty-nine weeks' gestation or later is medically indicated, induction for due dates alone is elective. A doctor saying "time's up" without a clear medical indication is coercive care that piles on risk—like painful contractions, infection, C-section, and uterine rupture.

Dozens of my survey respondents said their induction was the hardest part of birth. They cited the waiting, the pain, and the feeling of failure. "I really believed that my body failed," said Amanda in Denver. "During that induction I was confused and never understood why certain things were happening." She's describing a kind of imposter syndrome that can accompany induction, which a number of survey respondents alluded to. People felt ashamed that their bodies hadn't "done better" or had failed because birth didn't "start naturally." Many of the women surveyed said post-term pregnancy was "agony" and that doctors pressured them to induce or didn't give them a choice. Some didn't know they had one. Alison in Midvale, Utah, said four of her five children were born after their due date and that each time "it was hard to wait and to not feel pressured to induce." Teale in Annapolis, Maryland, was pressed to induce two of her births.

Elective induction has been steadily rising in frequency. In 1990, one out of every ten pregnant women were induced; by 2004 that number had jumped to one in five. By the time the third edition of the popular survey Listening to Mothers was published in 2013, 41 percent of mothers who gave birth in hospitals said their providers had tried to induce their labor. Inductions increased during the coronavirus pandemic, as providers convinced women that birth would be safer if it was turned on with a switch. But safer for whom? One Philadelphia hospital increased labor inductions from 36 to 42 percent in just three months. Can it be that close to half of women require drugs for labor to begin?

Absolutely not, was the response from researchers Jason Gardosi, Tracey Vanner, and Andy Francis, who examined more than twenty-four thousand hospital birth records and published their findings in the *British Journal of Obstetrics and Gynaecology* in 2005. They concluded that the majority of pregnancies induced for being "post-term" are actually not post-term at all when you look at their ultrasound dates; last menstrual period dates only give that false impression. "The proportion of pregnancies considered 'post-term' can be reduced considerably by a dating policy which ignores menstrual dates and establishes the expected delivery date on the basis of ultrasound dates alone," they wrote.

IT'S HARD TO IMAGINE PREGNANCY TODAY WITHOUT ULTRASOUND scans, which most pregnant people receive as their babies develop. Some women get one at every prenatal visit—which is as unnecessary as it is billable. The technology, which aims sound waves inaudible to humans at pregnant abdomens to create fetal images, was invented in the 1950s and widely adopted in England and America in the 1970s. It can be the most reliable method of dating a pregnancy when deployed at the right time. Experts say that the most accurate gestational age measurements are those based on ultrasounds done from weeks eleven to fourteen. Both ACOG and the Society for Maternal-Fetal Medicine say that doctors should use a combination of last menstrual period dates and early ultrasounds to come up with their "best estimate" for gestational age and a due date. They recommend that providers move due dates, once established, "only in rare circumstances." In fact, researchers found that women who received early ultrasound dating of their pregnancies were also less likely to be induced. Solely relying on the first day of the last menstrual period makes induction more likely.

Some pregnant people don't have access to routine ultrasound dating in the eleven-to-fourteen-week window. Some aren't getting the prenatal care they need at all. Black women are more likely than white women to lack insurance coverage at the start of pregnancies—sometimes they earn too much to qualify for Medicaid, but not enough to be able to afford other healthcare plans. The uninsured often forgo early prenatal care, meaning they miss the opportunity to establish a good due date. Without that ultrasound, though, dates are more likely to be wrong, and more likely to cause stress and unnecessary interventions later. This isn't women's fault. It's a systemic failure to recognize the need for these scans, to make them accessible to every pregnant person, and also to trust the pregnant person and physiologic labor process enough so as not to cling dramatically to a deadline for when labor must start *or else*. When doctors tell women they "won't let" them stay pregnant beyond a set number of weeks, and when women internalize the idea that they are not permitted to remain pregnant, that paternalism creates unnecessary pressure, anguish, and harm.

"We don't typically let women go beyond forty-two weeks," Copel told me.

The technology to date pregnancies using ultrasound has only existed for the past fifty years. Before that, there were fewer inductions and C-sections, and often more hands-on care. Copel remembers that when he was a medical student at Tufts University in the late 1970s, his job on the obstetrics rotation was to check for babies' heartbeats in first-trimester pregnant women. "We would listen and see if we could hear the heartbeat with a regular stethoscope, which happens at about eighteen weeks," he said. "And then they would come back every week until we could hear the heartbeat."

They also palpated the uterus externally with their hands to measure its size, something midwives have been doing for eons. "In the first trimester you can date a pregnancy just based on the size of the uterus from a manual exam," Copel said. Such methods take more time, but they offer more human connection, more hands-on care.

When I was pregnant with my third child, a provider recommended that I consider moving my due date back a week after analyzing my twelve-week ultrasound scan. The baby was measuring large, in keeping with a due date of August 20 rather than August 27, the date I had derived from the first day of my last menstrual period (a date I was pretty sure about). I consulted with my midwife, and she recommended that we stick with the original date, the 27th, but also to be ready if the baby decided to arrive earlier than that. I was grateful. I didn't want to feel pressure to birth, especially since I knew that a normal pregnancy length could vary by more than five weeks.

What's disconcerting but unsurprising is that none of the research on due dates and induction actually considers the preferences or experiences of birthing people themselves, according to the childbirth resource Evidence Based Birth. The one person whose final word matters most is ignored.

Considering all of the flaws and guesswork that estimating due dates entails, how should we think about them, and how should we use them? Due dates shouldn't be deadlines. Midwives advise pregnant people to think of their due dates as a window or a range instead of a specific day—more like a "due month." This revision might help alleviate external pressure from folks (bosses, mothers-in-law, etc.) who might worry and bother if a baby doesn't arrive on the promised schedule. As long as everyone is healthy and safe—which should be assumed unless there is good reason not to—why meddle? Why force a labor to start? I sometimes wonder what Sloane, Valerie, and Olivia would make of all this. If they someday decide to become pregnant, will they be pressured to induce based on misinterpretations of an ovulatory cycle that they weren't taught about?

It took me until my third pregnancy to think about birth this way. At that point, I began to really communicate it like this to colleagues, friends, and even strangers. When people asked me when I was due, I almost always said, "The end of August." If they pressed, sometimes I'd relent and specify the date with a qualifier: "But we know babies almost never arrive on their due dates. I don't expect this one to either."

In the end, my baby arrived very early on the morning of August 21. A few hours earlier and it would have been August 20, exactly the date my twelve-week ultrasound predicted. Naegele's method and the due date calculators were a week off. My baby was also enormous—nearly nine pounds. A speedster, growth-wise, and right on time.

THE NEXT PREGNANCY MILESTONE AFTER PROJECTING A DUE DATE is what I experienced when I spent days feeling on the verge of throwing up, without actually doing it. My gut sloshed like a washer full of clothes for the entirety of a cross-country flight for a story assignment. I picked up a rental car, then drove straight to TJ Maxx to buy a larger bra. Somehow, I'd outgrown the one I was wearing as we were flying over the desert. I ate stacks of saltine crackers, straight from tall plastic sleeves, and downed ginger candy and tea. I drove to my cousin's house where I burrowed myself into her couch. There I could fend off emails and try to sleep, the only time I wasn't miserable. Part of me wanted to just vomit already, get it over with. But vomiting didn't cure the terrible wrenching within. It was like a hand had reached inside and was trying to pull something out. Then my stomach would be empty and hungry and mad that bad crackers were all I could safely ingest.

Up to 90 percent of pregnant people experience what is commonly known as "morning sickness," a condition that ranges from manageable and mildly annoying to debilitating and potentially lethal. The first tell that this condition is minimized is the inaccurate and trivializing name we know it by. The timing suggestion is a misnomer, as the nausea can happen at any time, day or night. While for most people symptoms subside after the first trimester, the illness can persist for any duration.

The official name is nausea and vomiting of pregnancy (NVP). The most serious version is called hyperemesis gravidarum (HG). Kate,

Princess of Wales, was hospitalized with this; Charlotte Brontë is believed to have died from it. Not all who suffer are English—HG afflicts up to 3 percent of pregnancies. That's a low estimate; hardly all cases are counted. There's a high bar for suffering to secure a diagnosis. According to ACOG, a pregnant person may be diagnosed when she "has lost 5 percent of her pre-pregnancy body weight, and has other problems related to dehydration." She's not only failing to gain weight but actively losing it as her pregnancy progresses. Risk factors include previously experiencing the condition, being related to a woman who has had it, and, curiously, being pregnant with a female fetus. The treatment is mostly plunging IVs into arms to prevent dehydration and starvation. It's less a treatment than a measure to keep the sufferer alive.

Some degree of NVP plagues nearly all pregnant people. However, doctors frequently disbelieve women when they report how they feel. This is a nationwide problem. In Texas, one of my survey respondents, Ebony, reported that her doctor didn't believe her when she complained of severe symptoms that kept her from eating and gaining weight. "My doctor thought I was exaggerating," she said. Later, she learned that she should have been diagnosed with HG. She got it again in her second pregnancy and switched providers. In Wisconsin, Jennifer's doctor refused her medication. "I spent every single day of pregnancy vomiting with no relief," she said. Dalia in Quebec City was also ill for her entire pregnancy. In Minnesota, Becky's insurance company cut her off from treatment, indiscriminately capping how many pills she could have. Sonya, Kenyatta, and Tiffany said their nausea was by far the worst part of their pregnancies.

These examples are current, and yet they are rooted in a history of disbelieving and neglecting women's pain. An early theory about NVP described it as a psychological ailment that manifested as a physical one. In 1881, an obstetrician claimed he cured a woman of HG through psychiatric treatment. This assertion resonated for decades and was used to blame women for their own suffering. About one hundred years later, "underlying elements of emotional disturbance" were said to be found in severe cases. In the 1970s, when Sigmund

Freud's psychoanalytic theories seized the sciences and the larger culture, they became an undeniable influence in the diagnosis and treatment of women experiencing NVP. Women were neurotic when they
weren't pregnant; naturally, their craziness surged when they were.

Not only were sick pregnant women rejecting their pregnancies,
trying to dislodge fetuses by vomiting, they were also rebuffing sexual intercourse, their husbands, and the roles of motherhood and
womanhood, the thinking went. The apogee of their rejection of self
and place was the manifestation of physical illness. The vomiting was
thought to represent "a rejection of femininity or a rejection of pregnancy and impending motherhood via an unconscious, oral attempt
at abortion," explains the obstetrician Chavi Karkowsky in her book
High Risk.

An outgrowth of this theory was the belief that women were faking suffering to gain attention. A 1971 gynecology text warned that
"many women, wittingly or unwittingly, exaggerate the severity of
their complaints to gratify neurotic desires." Doctors practicing today
learned this in medical school. Their textbooks, mentors, and predecessors told stories of women's unruly bodies and unhinged minds.
Even if doctors would never cop to believing this, it would have been a
difficult portrayal to avoid during their training.

Karkowsky, who treats patients with severe HG, says there are typically a couple of patients suffering from the condition during every
shift she works. "When I look now at the application of the psychiatric explanation and resulting treatments of Nausea and Vomiting of
Pregnancy, the total effect seems to be one of enormous amounts of
anger directed at pregnant women suffering from these conditions,"
she wrote. When NVP and HG are "invented mental problems," it
becomes acceptable to both "dismiss women's suffering" and "blame
them for it."

Perhaps a generous interpretation of why we blame victims of NVP
and HG is because of misplaced frustration that we don't know their
real cause. ACOG's FAQ about the conditions doesn't include one
question or answer about why they occur. There are theories: growing a new organ, the placenta, requires an infusion of hormones that

may cause queasiness; or perhaps it's adaptive, a sickness that prevents the pregnant woman from ingesting toxins or engaging in dangerous activities that could harm the fetus. But we don't in fact know what causes these ailments.

And that's the point. Plenty of medical practitioners don't believe that it's important to know. Why work to discover a mostly short-lived problem's source? Sure, the majority of pregnant people suffer from it to some degree. But for most it's relatively mild and gone in a few months.

Existing medications can alleviate the worst symptoms. But I've spoken to many mothers who had to ask for them repeatedly or were not offered them at all. Instead, doctors suggested they eat ginger and saltine crackers, like I did, and eliminate spicy foods. Only after she had tried this and remained in agony for months did one friend's doctor finally, begrudgingly, alert her that there were stronger remedies like vitamin B6, and both over-the-counter and prescriptions drugs. "Why didn't you tell me sooner? Why did I have to be sick for weeks and then ask again?" she wondered.

When Karkowsky was pregnant, she had to write her own prescription for medication to treat her debilitating NVP after her own obstetrician would not. She suspects that for many women "the misery persists because the medical establishment still doesn't value the suffering of the mother over the smallest possible risk to her growing fetus." This, when the remedies are virtually risk-free.

WELCOME TO PREGNANCY. YOU RECEIVE A DUE DATE BASED ON A menstrual cycle that didn't happen. Surprise: it's the day your doctor will later pressure or force you to give birth! Next, you're sick with an illness so common that no one cares, so underexamined that its cause is a mystery, and, because you're a woman, you might even be disbelieved, mocked, or blamed for your suffering. Treatment will also likely be withheld. Then, you're plunged into a sea of decisions about procedures and tests and choices about the people with whom and the place in which you'll birth. Afraid yet?

Despite the major stroller presence in their neighborhood, Sloane, Valerie, and Olivia know none of this. I didn't even acknowledge my pregnancy with them until the end of our conversation. I wanted to listen to them, not talk about me. I did when they finally felt tentative permission to ask me about it. They had wondered about the mechanics—how penises fit into vaginas and how babies got out. Olivia's mom had told them once, at breakfast, that vaginas are very stretchy. Was this true? I told them it was. They asked if pregnancy made me feel sick. I said a little in the beginning but not anymore.

CHAPTER 2
FEAR OF DEATH

BEN AND I ARE HAVING DINNER WITH FRIENDS AT A FAVORITE spot, where the hanging plants keep multiplying and you can try any wine you want. We met through our kids. When John's wife gave birth, doctors used forceps and a vacuum.

"She labored and pushed, and the baby just wouldn't come out," he says. A plate of octopus parts sits between us, the small protuberances glistening. I usually conceal my disdain for the abuse people endure but don't always recognize as they have their babies. But in this setting tonight, I'm a little freer with my criticism of how childbirth happens. Maybe that's why John is more forthcoming about the details of his wife's birth, his fear and horror as it occurred. I'm letting slip what I usually don't say—that too often doctors' routine interventions are abuse, that either they don't know how birth works or don't adequately support it. Is this information people want to hear? He nods, but I can see the words sting, maybe rankle. Now he must convince me of the indispensability of the treatment she received. Of his gratitude.

"It was really scary," he tells me. We're sitting outside and an overhead heater is making us sweat. He says his wife's experiences were exceptions. She, the baby—the entire family, really—needed the technology, the intervention. They're glad it happened. Relieved.

"I'm grateful for hospitals and doctors," John says with a smile that's both pleading and pained. "They probably saved her life and our baby's life."

Before I gave birth, I struggled to believe the act was possible. I saw ultrasound photos of a skeletal form; I was unconvinced that it would become folds of flesh, pink gums, hair. It was a terrifying act of faith, much like the choice to parent, that something alive and that I would instantly love could emerge from a place typically rendered unspeakable.

As I reached the life stage when the women around me started to give birth—first colleagues, then friends—they shared the fact of it, but that was both start and finish. I read the birth announcement emails authored by proud partners. The sappy, grateful social media posts. I scanned the photos for parents in hairnets, partners in scrubs—tells of the surgical birth hidden from the pronouncement. These dispatches assured that mom and baby were "resting well" or "recovering smoothly," divulged baby names and statistics, swooned about new parenthood, and joked about the lack of sleep. But they said nothing about what I really hungered to know: What was it like? What *actually* happened during childbirth?

The stories leaked out when we were face-to-face. Galina had an emergency C-section, she told me, after her baby's "heart rate dropped." Kendel had one too, after endless hours of laboring and pushing. The anesthesiologist at the hospital where Susan both worked and gave birth botched her epidural. Her subsequent crushing headaches and dizziness came from a spinal fluid leak. Madhu was left alone in post-op for four hours, waiting for an orderly to take her to a recovery room, while her partner and family spent time with the baby; she believed she was purposely kept apart from them, when in fact she had been forgotten. Doctors diagnosed Alex, during the births of both of her children, with failure to progress and performed two emergency C-sections, the second of which she believed was "avoidable." I'm not sure how a procedure can be both an emergency and avoidable. Rachel believes that her C-section saved her life. So does Priya.

Are lives routinely saved during childbirth? The narrative we know insists that they are, that childbirth is dangerous, that hospitals are safe. Becoming pregnant myself, I marveled at the bounty of people I knew whose labors had suddenly, without warning, become calamitous. Cords encircling necks, plummeting heart rates, stalled progress, stuck babies. I hardly ever heard a birth story that was powerful or easy, or even just vaginal, with no interventions. Every uterus needed kick-starting with a chemical induction. Every labor was too long; every birth was a crisis. Every baby was in danger inside and was better off outside, their first home suddenly inhospitable. Women became risks to their babies, to themselves. What I observed, that birth was always an emergency, started to seem normal. It took years of reporting—and giving birth myself three times—to realize how insane that is.

Neel Shah has gone to the grocery store or the dog park, still in his scrubs, with a fleece jacket over them announcing his job: OBGYN. "Someone finds out in the real world what I do for a living, they will often spontaneously tell me their birth story," the obstetrician and Harvard professor tells me. The tales are not mundane and usually involve heroism: a doctor saving a mom's or baby's life. "If they have had a C-section, they'll usually tell me a story where in my head I'm thinking, 'Man, that's not why you had a C-section.' They're like, 'Oh, my baby's cord was wrapped around his neck and, you know, they saved his life.' And in my head, I'm thinking, 'We deliver babies with their cord wrapped around their necks vaginally all the time. It's not even a sometimes thing.'"

Women and their families often leave their births thinking that interventions saved their babies' lives or their own lives. That they needed drugs, cuts, shots, and operations for everyone to survive. "In most cases, when women have had a C-section, their understanding of what happened to them is really different from what clinicians' understanding would be," Shah says. He calls this chasm between truth and fiction "a tragedy."

It's impossible to know what percentage of people believe that interventions performed during their childbirths were lifesaving. Interventions like inducing labor with manufactured prostaglandins, quickening contractions with synthetic oxytocin, and numbing the body with an epidural steroid injection can cause labors to stall and heart rates to drop, inviting a trip to the OR. One thing is certain, however, during childbirth: fear.

THE BIRTH DANGER PARABLE SNAKES THROUGH OUR CELEBRATED literature and through popular television shows and films. In *War and Peace*, Princess Lise gives birth in a cacophony of screams, then inexplicably dies. Leo Tolstoy implies that birth is reason enough to succumb, as he gives no other cause. Catherine Earnshaw, the tormented antihero of Emily Brontë's *Wuthering Heights*, passes after giving birth to her daughter. Agnes of Mudfog dies when Oliver Twist is born. At the end of Gabriel García Márquez's *One Hundred Years of Solitude*, not only does Amaranta Úrsula die, but her child is eaten by ants, fulfilling the curse of the Buendía family's erasure. The entire world of *Game of Thrones*, the most watched show to air on premium television, is erected on the bodies of dead mothers. More than a dozen people die in the birthing bed during the eight-season series, but the centerpiece of the plot is Joanna Lannister's death when Tyrion is born.

Narratively speaking, the death of a birth mother often serves a male central character. It softens a fickle persona, excuses brash behavior, and creates luscious complexity in an otherwise flat plot. On the mega-popular Netflix series *Bridgerton*, Simon Basset is a cruel sex object until we learn of his mother's death while giving birth to him, the family heir, whom she doesn't live long enough to hold. In this moment he becomes human, sympathetic.

Mothers dead from childbirth are perhaps the original set

piece—conveniently normalized and accepted by audiences. This plot device detonates female characters in service of elevating and humanizing adjacent men. Her tragic exit is the start of his hero's journey.

When characters habitually die giving birth, a lie is told about birth. Here, it is not ultimate power but common peril. Birth unearths her inherent weakness. Giving life so easily kills her. Her death is what makes him (it's almost always him) come alive. Adrienne Rich writes that this is a product of who's in charge: "Typically in patriarchy the mother's life is exchanged for the child." It's difficult to witness this so often in the cultural cannon and not let it seep in. These fictional childbirth deaths subconsciously haunt us. When we inure ourselves to them in entertainment, we believe that they are common in life too.

They are not.

In the US, hundreds die from childbirth each year out of about four million births. The losses are also unjust, especially as they are more likely to occur when birthers are Black and Brown and because childbirth deaths are largely preventable. But it's a small number compared to, say, car deaths, of which there are about forty thousand each year on American roads. Most of us drive every day, and few of us experience any trepidation doing so. We're not afraid to enter our cars, but somehow we live in morbid fear of pushing a human from between our legs.

The global maternal mortality rate is hard to parse, as it masks important nuances and differences. But it has been declining since the 1990s, according to a 2021 report from the Bill & Melinda Gates Foundation. America's rate—thirty-five deaths for every one hundred thousand births—is an order of magnitude higher than that of other countries where midwifery care is common and where home birth is a choice you can make while remaining part of the healthcare system. In Canada the rate is eight; in western Europe, it's five; in Australia, two.

When birth killed one in forty women in medieval Europe, we hadn't yet discovered bacteria. We didn't know that hand washing was lifesaving. It was typical for a woman to produce a dozen children, and without knowledge of or access to reliable birth control or proper pregnancy spacing, some bodies succumbed. People died giving birth. But the narrative that birth was historically dangerous and regularly deadly contradicts evidence of good outcomes in childbirth.

Records of birth in Puritan England and in the American colonies reveal that midwife-attended childbirths were very successful. As the colonies grew, birth became even safer in America than in the crowded cities of Europe, where diseases traveled easily before the advent of antimicrobial drugs and routine hand washing, with better survival rates for both mothers and infants. In colonial New England, "childbearing, while a danger, has been overestimated as a cause of death," according to historians Richard and Dorothy Wertz, authors of the academic social history of childbirth *Lying-in*. One historian they cite found that "if all the women in seventeenth-century Plymouth who died during childbearing years died because of birth complications, birth was still successful 95 percent of the time."

A maternal death rate of about half a percent was typical in late eighteenth- to early nineteenth-century America, according to birth records. This was "miniscule" compared to the era's perceptions, writes Jacqueline Wolf in *Deliver Me from Pain: Anesthesia and Birth in America*, though it would be high today. Historians believe the fear of dying in childbirth was "exaggerated" and attributable "to the belief that labor pain was just punishment meted out by God, a principle conveyed and reinforced by the predominant religion," Wolf explains. The high number of births experienced by eighteenth- and nineteenth-century women, alongside repeated stories of death, amplified fears. Actual death in childbirth was far less common than the fear of it.

Still, that birth is inherently hazardous to mothers and babies is perhaps the primary belief that shapes how humans are born today. We birth the way we do because we fear it. This fear is not inevitable. It is created and learned. And the male doctors who usurped control of childbirth in twentieth-century America both manipulated and amplified it.

FOR MOST OF HUMAN HISTORY, BABIES ARRIVED EXCLUSIVELY IN the company of women. A mother labored among female friends, neighbors, and family members. Childbirth was ritual and celebration, a rarefied time to sideline domestic work, coalesce support, and enshrine female bonds. Birth reigned as the "fundamental occasion for the expression of care and love among women" in early America, according to the Wertzes.

The women assisted the midwife with tasks—applying compresses, preparing food, holding the laborer's body. Their payment was appreciation and reciprocity; women who attended birth would have their birth supported in return. By the time girls became women, they had aided so much childbirth that it was well-known territory. Being integral to these births likely eliminated some of the fear of doing it. Social childbirth, as this was called, has disappeared in America. Today, the first and only childbirth most pregnant people witness is their own.

Recently, I received a Paperless Post invite to a Zoom "Blessing Way" for a pregnant mom. The invitation credited the Navajo tradition with the custom, a prebirth gathering of a pregnant person's most trusted women friends and family members. There are books about how to throw a Blessing Way, or "mother-centered baby shower." Each guest was asked to mail a small bead, which the future mother would thread on a necklace to wear during her labor. The necklace would embody the women who loved her. Then they could be with her, in spirit if not in flesh. That was the idea anyway. At the Zoom Blessing Way, people hoisted the beads they were giving the new mom up to the cameras on their screens and chronicled their attendant qualities—a cleansing amethyst, a strength-giving tiger's eye. The idea of the necklace was tender and thoughtful; I briefly wished I had known to ask for this ahead of my births. Learning birth's history as a woman-led sacrament, though, I also wonder why we accept that a necklace could be enough.

We aren't physically present for each other during our childbirths anymore. Instead of filling our homes with the motions and sounds of ritual, with the hand-holding service of people who love us, we travel to a place we've never been before and entrust our bodies to strangers in uniform who hold professional degrees. More recently, maximalist Covid-19 restrictions ensured that fewer supporters were allowed in birth wards: doulas, mothers, sisters, and even partners were banned in the name of protecting medical staff. Some hospitals continue to forbid doulas access to their clients' births even as the pandemic has abated. It's hard to think of something more frightening, more upsetting than being forced to birth alone. The only thing more distressing, perhaps, is the irrational fear of dying while giving birth. After all, birth wasn't designed to be dangerous. A mother's body isn't a weapon aimed at the baby it creates, or vice versa. A successful birth—mom and baby thriving—is nature's preference.

Birth in America became more dangerous when men began attending it instead of women.

MIDWIFERY WAS MEDICINE'S FIRST PROFESSIONAL GAMBIT IN America, the Wertzes explain. But not the midwifery of Indigenous and immigrant women, passed down through generations of apprentices. The first men to attend birth learned the trade from women midwives, then called what they were doing "the new midwifery" to distinguish themselves.

When medical colleges began to spring up in the United States to professionalize healing in the mid- to late eighteenth century, the first specialty they taught was "midwifery," as it was assumed to be "a keystone to medical practice, something that every student would do after graduation." If delivering babies was fundamental to medicine, men, the only people allowed to practice, wanted to deliver babies to be considered serious doctors. Men believed this ancient work was "new" because they were doing it.

Professionalizing medicine meant convincing communities to discard traditional knowledge and methods of care. Social birth was disbanded, and midwife-led networks were broken up. "The triumph of the male medical profession involved the destruction of women's networks of mutual help—leaving women in a position of isolation and dependency," write Barbara Ehrenreich and Deirdre English in *For Her Own Good: Two Centuries of the Experts' Advice to Women*. Ancestral knowledge was rebranded as ignorance. The patience that midwives had exhibited was dismissed as ignorance, and the comfort measures they provided were labeled outmoded, slow, and unclean. The necessary ritual was recast as antiquated.

Men professionalized birth work through the development of the obstetrics field, which evolved to look very different from the supportive birth Indigenous and immigrant midwives offered. For starters, they manufactured a narrative to undergird this development: that birth guided by midwives was dangerous and uncouth, whereas birth directed by male doctors was safe and preserved modesty.

In the Victorian era—that of pregnancy corsets and fainting couches—the medical field's intrusion into childbirth coincided with a rise in ideas of women's femininity and purity. Women longed for a way to be ushered into motherhood that was safe, comfortable, and quick. They wanted men to care for them, to witness and validate their pain, the Wertzes wrote. Male doctors were the natural "guardians of female modesty" and the "indispensable comforters of women," the same as "guardian with ward, father with daughter, priest and confessee." The power dynamic was desired by women and doctors alike. Women were afraid; they believed that being shepherded and controlled was necessary for their safety and self-actualization. It was a kind of "moral therapy," ensuring not only "less painful and unsafe births" but also "a generally happier, more fulfilling life." Not all women chose this path for themselves, of course; some were surely forced into the position of supplicant or swayed by cultural expectations of modesty. However, the story of heroic doctors aided a male takeover of birth. By extension, male doctors furthered the notion that labor itself was dangerous and that women were too fragile to withstand it. Roll out the fainting couch.

Belief in women's frailty in the face of childbirth persisted into the twentieth century. "The powers of natural labor are dangerous and destructive to mother and child," Joseph DeLee, the obstetrician and founder of the Chicago Lying-in Hospital, explained to his colleagues in the American Gynecological Society in 1921. "Interference by a skilled accoucheur at the proper time can prevent a goodly portion of this danger and much of this destruction." DeLee was articulating a theory growing in popularity: Natural childbirth was inherently dangerous. It paralyzed women with fear and rendered them helpless and unable to perform its taxing, physical work. Breathing through contractions, slowing down, stretching the perineum gradually—all this and more was beyond women's abilities, DeLee said.

With this framing, he "breathed life into what we know as modern obstetrics," writes Jennifer Block, author of the childbirth history *Pushed*. DeLee manifested the type of childbirth necessary for obstetrics to exist. The birth he championed and standardized was one spawned by the medical arts, as this new tool use was called, rather than the one perfected over eons by evolution. DeLee claimed that physiologic birth—the process women's bodies naturally undergo—was actually treacherous for them and that they would be safer and emerge even better from the ordeal by letting their bodies be medicated and operated on.

DeLee's "The Prophylactic Forceps Operation" speech was later reprinted in the *American Journal of Obstetrics and Gynecology*, where it became a rubric for how an obstetrician could birth a baby *for* someone. It advocated for a transfer of generative power from birthers to doctors and tabulated the necessary steps. First, administer morphine and scopolamine, then ether; next, cut the nerves, muscles, and tissues of the perineum, remove the baby with forceps, and stitch up the episiotomy; finally, dose round two of morphine and scopolamine "to prolong narcosis for many hours postpartum, and to abolish the memory of the labor as much as possible." This tool-produced (read: drugged and manipulated) birth would imbue the obstetrics profession with even more status and credibility.

DeLee and like-minded colleagues wielded this theory and practice to argue for abolishing midwives and replacing them with obstetricians, a plan they would effectively execute over subsequent decades. Ehrenreich and English likened the effort to how Nazis exterminated Jews: "The American medical profession would settle for nothing less than the final solution to the midwife question: they would have to be eliminated—outlawed."

After first studying with midwives, then directly competing with them, male obstetricians finally forced them from birth work with laws, codes, courts, required schooling, regulations, and ultimately hospital systems that banned them. To practice midwifery in a hospital setting today requires a nursing degree.

Midwives didn't bow to their competition. They attacked with tools and tongues. One pro-midwifery broadside describing the emergence of obstetrics said that "Satan vomited up a set of reptiles calling themselves midwife-doctors." But midwives weren't as organized as doctors and couldn't strategically mount a fight. They apprenticed to learn their skills; they didn't professionalize or institutionalize their craft. Their expertise wasn't book bound. It was (and is) the doing kind.

Notably, they also lacked organized feminist support. This was in no small part because midwives were most often immigrants and people of color. Middle-class, white activist women supported women who looked like them becoming medical school students and doctors rather than fighting to preserve the expertise of immigrant midwives, who were described by their opponents as "hopelessly dirty, ignorant, and incompetent." Access to the white male world of medicine proved more desirable than protecting what women traditionally did and knew.

Between 1900 and 1930, midwives "were almost totally eliminated," Ehrenreich and English explain, outlawed across states and attacked or undermined by local authorities. And banning women from obstetrics and midwifery "gave obstetrics a sexist bias; maleness became a necessary attribute for safety, and femaleness became a condition in need of male medical control," the Wertzes write. In 1930 the American Board of Obstetrics and Gynecology was created, further walling off the profession to outsiders, like midwives.

In the process of medicalizing birth, men relocated labor and delivery to hospitals. At the turn of the twentieth century, only 5 percent of babies were born in hospitals. By 1921, the same year that DeLee gave his persuasive speech to the American Gynecological Society, hospitals accounted for more than half of all births in major American cities. People had been successfully convinced they were safer there. The new setting did two important things. First, it allowed the medical profession to transform obstetrics into a science concerned with the physical processes of birth, rather than with the person doing it.

Second, it ensured the privacy for doctors to do what they wanted to patients, as women's families weren't allowed inside treatment rooms. Tools such as forceps became important, as doctors needed technology to prove their worth, their fees, and their prowess. Male birth attendants, too impatient "to sit around for hours watching a hole," as one doctor put it, interceded, endangering women.

"If labor was too slow for his schedule he intervened with knife or forceps, often to the detriment of mother or child," according to Ehrenreich and English. At teaching hospitals, doctors trained students in surgical interventions because they wanted them to be able to perform them in rare, complicated cases. Waiting for a normal birth didn't fit into the program: it was too slow and didn't require their tools. Thus, laboring women and their families came to expect speedier deliveries with the aid of "modern medicine." Today, obstetric residents are exposed to more surgical births than vaginal ones.

The birth procedure that DeLee prescribed became the norm as childbirth moved from homes to hospitals in the early twentieth century. And in hospitals, childbearers began to mingle with disease sufferers. Infection became the greatest threat to the expectant mother, as germ theory, which had existed for some time, still hadn't been fully incorporated into medical practice. Doctors didn't routinely wash their hands. Death among birthers increased. Wealthy women were more likely to die, as they could afford doctors and hospitals. Poor women, who still used midwives, were spared.

The dominant cause of death postpartum in the nineteenth and into the twentieth century was puerperal fever, typically originating from a placental infection. One Philadelphia doctor, who saw ninety-five cases in his practice in four years, reported eighteen of them as fatal. Some 75 percent of patients at Boston's lying-in hospital contracted the ailment, and 20 percent died of it, in 1883. By 1934, hospital infection rates were still as high as 11 percent. Negligence in disinfectant practices only fueled puerperal fever, which continued to infect and kill birthers until the 1940s.

Oliver Wendell Holmes, a dean at Harvard Medical School, attributed its contagion to doctors spreading it from patient to patient in the mid-1800s, but he was ignored and dismissed. "God only knows the number of women whom I have consigned prematurely to the grave," said physician Ignaz Philipp Semmelweis in Vienna, who proved around the same time that hand washing eliminated puerperal fever, but not before he had caused untold death. Few of his colleagues believed him, however, and he was fired. Later, he was committed to a psychiatric hospital.

The Wertzes call puerperal fever "the classic example of iatrogenic disease—disease that is caused by medical treatment itself." They believe that it's "useless" to speculate about whether midwives would have sickened and killed fewer birthers than doctors, even though they were less likely to carry bacteria, operate, and apply unsterilized tools, because "the basis of comparison is missing."

In 1933, a report from the White House Conference on Child Health and Protection revealed that maternal mortality rose in the "great migration" to hospital birth that took place between 1915 and 1929. Infant deaths skyrocketed during roughly the same period, increasing by between 40 and 50 percent in data drawn from eleven states. The report offered two reasons for the mortality hike: absent or inadequate prenatal care and "excessive intervention" in birth, "often improperly performed." An investigation of maternal mortality in New York found that two-thirds of the more than two thousand deaths could have been prevented "had the best medical knowledge been applied."

As a point of comparison from a few decades later, Margaret Charles Smith, a Black midwife in rural Alabama, attended some three thousand births in homes between 1949 and 1981 without a single mother dying. The 2006 book *Listen to Me Good: The Life Story of an Alabama Midwife* documents her career serving Black women like herself "whose lives, by her own account, were not being lived in an environment that led to good health."

It wasn't birth that was killing people. It was men and hospitals.

By the 1940s and 1950s, it had become impossibly clear that doctors themselves were causing puerperal fever. Many sounded alarms, and the plague ended. But strategies to save lives had the ancillary effect of further dehumanizing hospital birth. The discovery and then fear of germs led hospital staff to shave women's pubic hair, clean their torsos with ether, shampoo their heads using kerosene, and douche them with saline and whiskey. This routine would later be found to spread new diseases that assaulted hospitals and that doctors were trying to fight. Meanwhile, DeLee's prophylactic forceps operation gained reputation as superior and became standardized. This technique allowed doctors to leave patients alone for hours and hours, only showing up to administer drugs and operate. Thus, well into the twentieth century, women continued to "be processed as possibly diseased objects," withstanding horrendous treatment as they brought new life into the world.

It was mostly kept quiet that routine birth had become barbaric in the name of preventing death and disease. That changed in 1957, when a labor and delivery nurse wrote a letter published in the *Ladies' Home Journal*, exhorting authorities to start an investigation into what she called "cruelty in maternity wards." Hundreds of women replied to share how they had been "dehumanized" during birth. Some had been strapped down like "trapped animals" for days at a time.

"For 36 hours my husband didn't know whether I was living or dead," wrote one woman. A veterinarian's wife said she had been treated like a circus sideshow; dogs and cats, she noted, received better care when giving birth. A third woman, who had given birth in three hospitals with three different doctors, concluded, "Women are herded like sheep through an obstetrical assembly line, are drugged and strapped on tables while their babies are forceps-delivered. Obstetricians today are businessmen who run baby factories. Modern painkillers and methods are used for the convenience of the doctor, not to spare the mother."

AFTER A HUNDRED YEARS OF PROFESSIONALIZED MEDICINE, women have internalized doctors' control over their bodies during birth as inevitable. If something goes wrong, it's never the doctor's fault. "Women would rather have the experience of trying everything, of the doctor saying we did everything we could, than risk something going wrong and blaming themselves," Lisa Rubin, associate professor of psychology at the New School, told me. What she says makes infinite sense. If doctors don't "do everything" and something does go wrong, women think ahead to the blame they'll feel. They will fault themselves for "not letting the doctors try everything."

Birthers have so thoroughly accepted doctors' control over their own bodies as natural that they even blame themselves for trauma inflicted on them. My survey showed a strong correlation between reporting birth trauma and feeling blamed or judged. We believe trauma is our fault when it is not, and we choose powerlessness over the potential for self-blame. I'm not sure whether this is a conscious choice. I do know that, no matter what kind of birth a woman has, she must give the thing a narrative to make sense of her loss of control— and overwhelmingly that narrative involves guilt. "I should have put my foot down more," said Allie, about her second C-section, which she had hoped would be a VBAC, a vaginal birth after cesarean. "That was my chance."

"Sometimes I felt that my three unconscious deliveries were yet another sign of my half-suspended inadequacy as a woman," wrote Adrienne Rich in 1976. "The 'real' mothers were those who had been 'awake through it all.'"

Rich's assertion is nearly fifty years old but dovetails with a contemporary reality: our desire to defend interventions we received but didn't want, while feeling imposter syndrome for not birthing naturally, the way we believe women *should*.

Like school or the office, birth is another societal opportunity for women to perform, to prove they're good girls. We can participate willingly or unwittingly in our own subjugation. Becoming patients, we are easily anonymized in stale gowns, our bodies filling rows of identical mechanical beds. When we are instructed, we obey. We do the thing because we believe that we should but also because we fear being trouble. It's too easy to be categorized as disobedient or difficult.

We assume the person telling us knows what he's talking about, that this is what other pregnant or laboring people have done, must do. We also worry for our personal safety and the well-being of our babies. If we don't listen, there could be life-altering consequences. After all, we are in a hospital. This is where disease and tragedy live, but also courage and miracles. We listen to others and not our bodies. They have no authority, no currency to purchase power in this society. We've spent our lives disconnected from them, tuning out their needs. Why would birth be the moment this changes?

CHAPTER 3
FEAR OF PAIN

WHEN I LEARNED I WAS PREGNANT WITH MY FIRST CHILD, I PRE-
sumed I'd have a hospital birth. Well, first I texted my husband
an image of the positive pregnancy test. Then I worried, briefly, about
the impact of having steeped myself (and my fetus) in Albariño and
unpasteurized Manchego during a recent trip to Barcelona. Next, I
stripped in front of a mirror, trying to conjure what my bare stomach
would look like when it swelled.

I envisioned sitting on a gurney in a papery gown, infant bundled
in the standard-issue pink-and-blue-striped blanket and pressed to my
chest. I believed that if I could learn enough about birth and choose
the right location and providers, that I could curate the birth experience I wanted, the beautiful entry into motherhood that I designed. It
was a privileged assumption. It was also wrong.

Both my mother and mother-in-law had avoided epidurals. I assumed that was what it meant to choose a natural birth. My mom

told me about delivering my brother in Atlanta in the mid-1980s, when the nurses came from different floors to lay eyes on the woman who had refused labor drugs. But didn't it hurt? I asked her. It must have hurt.

I picked up two primary sources on birth for a certain type of curious millennial: the book *Ina May's Guide to Childbirth* and a 2008 documentary, *The Business of Being Born*. Midwife author Ina May Gaskin and the team behind the documentary differ in their approaches but essentially draw the same conclusions: Birth is unlike anything you've ever done, but you can do it. A lot of women before you have. That's why you're even here.

In *The Business of Being Born*, I saw Ricki Lake welcome her child in a bathtub. For the first time, I could visualize a real alternative to the hospital: home birth, its polar opposite. I had first heard about home birth years earlier from a friend whose wife had just had a baby. At the time, I was freshly out of college and very far from that world. When I asked where his baby was born, and he said in our bathtub, I frowned. My first thought was that something must have gone haywire with the pregnancy, that the baby had come unexpectedly. But the look on his face was serene.

We wanted it, he said. It was awesome. She did great.

I wanted to know more about what it was like but didn't want to pry. I also secretly wondered whether she was crazy. Wasn't that a huge risk? Or maybe she knew something I didn't. I landed on crazy, mostly to bolster the choice I thought I would one day make. Now I was on the brink of making it.

I did consider a home birth with my first pregnancy. But every time I brought up home birth with friends or family members, they said it sounded dangerous. I disagreed with them, but their opinions assaulted my subconscious. I began to think my home wasn't the right location for childbirth. Did the act that bridged life and death, whose supposed pain was legendary, really belong in the place where I plucked hair from the drain, where I dragged a razor over my legs? I didn't fear dying. But I worried for my baby and dreaded torturous pain. Hospitals had the drugs.

The door to home birth was ajar; fear kicked it shut.

Instead, I interviewed doulas as protection against something going wrong. The dominant cultural message was very much that it would. I researched top-tier neonatal intensive-care units (NICUs), not C-section or episiotomy rates. My first prenatal visit was with a midwife in a fancy neighborhood. She sighed as I asked questions and bruised my arm doing routine bloodwork. I settled on another midwifery practice that delivered exclusively in the hospital closest to my home.

My plan was the best of both worlds—midwife-assisted birth exactly how I wanted it, with the backup of lifesaving technology and pain management at the ready, should I need them. Once I chose the practice attached to the hospital, I thought more judgmentally about home birth. I otherized it as scary, unsafe, painful. A perfect choice for any birther who felt it was perfect for her—but not the choice for me.

Perhaps no other gambit describes transitioning to motherhood more than the tendency to judge others' choices to reinforce our own. It feels less nefarious than necessary.

Meanwhile, my belly grew bigger as I anticipated the day baby would come.

MOST BOOKS FRAME BIRTH NOT AS A PROCESS IN THE BODY BUT A procedure in a hospital. A common hospital birth begins with a doctor unnecessarily administering a drug to start contractions. Next comes rupturing the bag of water, giving an epidural, and finally, after determining that labor has failed to progress, when the birthing person's body probably wasn't ready to go into labor to begin with, ordering abdominal surgery. More than half of us receive synthetic oxytocin, Pitocin, to speed up contractions to a level that can be so painful that we then need numbing below the waist with an epidural to tolerate them. A third of us—around 1.3 million Americans every year—give birth through abdominal surgery. "C-section is the first thing we all learn," an obstetrician told me. "They teach it to us when we're interns. This is the first birth case you learn. Any OBGYN. That's what they can do."

After a few visits to the midwife during my first pregnancy, it became clear that I didn't know what actually happened during childbirth and that nobody was going to explain it to me. I noticed how birth conversation, no matter whom it was with, centered on the hospital and what went on there. What to put in the bag you bring, what to buy, which tests to take while you're pregnant, what to eat or drink (or avoid)—but nothing about what happens when the body goes into labor. I wondered whether my body would go into labor on its own. What happened during a contraction, during a push? And what was I to do to manage the sensation of contraction? To cope with what would surely be unimaginable pain?

I wanted to meet my fear with facts. I found explanations in *Natural Childbirth the Bradley Way* by Susan McCutcheon. The book was published in 1984 and revised in 1996, and even though I was giving birth in 2015, reading it felt revelatory. It describes a method of childbirth created by an obstetrician named Robert Bradley that embraces the natural physiological process of childbirth, emphasizes the avoidance of medication and intervention, and teaches the practice of partners coaching. This book turned out to also be the companion text to the birthing class I took with Ben.

What I learned was that the muscular sack of the uterus holds and nurtures the growing fetus. Part sea creature, it bobs in a microcosmic ocean. The umbilical cord connects the baby to its life source, the placenta, an organ that the mother's body creates. It is the only example, in fact, of an adult human body making an organ. The placenta functions as the baby's heart, lungs, liver, digestive system, food source, waste remover, and regulatory system. In German, the placenta is called *Mutterkuchen*, or "mother cake," the nourisher. Baby blooms through a variety of fruit and vegetable sizes, to use the vernacular of pregnancy apps. When baby starts to require more resources than the placenta can supply, the uterus begins to contract, squeezing its considerable musculature to force open the cervix (Latin for neck). The cervix is made up of muscles powerful enough to keep uterine contents inside until the second they must be emptied. At that point, they pull open the cervix door and usher the baby downward. That's what we feel when the uterus contracts.

The midwife Ina May Gaskin imagines the uterus as a soft purse and the cervix as its gathered opening. Throughout a pregnancy, thick mucus seals shut the cervix door. As labor approaches, the cervical muscle ripens, or becomes flat and soft, losing its neck shape. The mucus thins so the plug it has formed will dislodge. Sometimes the plug frees along with blood, a signpost that labor will begin.

Gaskin describes the birthing person's mood as "restless" during this phase of intensity. The baby is being jostled into the optimal position. For humans, it's head first, but feet first and bottom first are also possible vaginally. Gravity aids birth. Abdominal pressure combines with uterine contractions to eventually birth the baby, then expel the placenta, whose job is done.

This is the physiology, but there are actions and environments that support or thwart it.

ROBERT BRADLEY GREW UP ON A FARM WATCHING ALL MANNER OF animals quietly birth their young. Witnessing the process convinced him of the ability and agency of the birthing body—bovine or human. He decided these bodies should be left alone, except for the care of a trusted, loving support person. A coach. Bradley started teaching husbands how to be good coaches during their wives' births in the 1950s. The objective was for the husband to guide his wife through medication- and intervention-free deliveries. He was among the first doctors in the country to bring husbands into the birth space; historically they had even been barred if not banned. The Bradley Method organization has since swapped the word *husband* for *partner* in many of its materials, since birth support people are not all married men.

Western culture assumes that birth requires a separation of the body from the mind—"thoughts and feelings are considered irrelevant to physical well-being and bodily functions," according to Gaskin. However, during birth, the two are intertwined. "True words spoken can sometimes relax pelvic muscles by discharging emotions that effectively block further progress in labor," she writes. At one birth she attended, a husband repeatedly told his wife she was "mar-velous." The woman believed that the words opened her cervix and invited the baby out.

Bradley understood this too. He said that birthing bodies need six things. Zero of them are available in hospitals.

The first is *darkness and solitude*. Bright lights disrupt concentration. Concentration is key to relaxation. It's hard to do either with hot lights blazing in your face. Solitude dovetails with this—being alone in the dark, or with a partner or support person, helps with concentration and relaxation.

"It is very distracting for most women to have observers during the first stage of labor," as McCutcheon put it. Observers turn the first stage of labor into a performance. When you feel like you have to put on a show, it's tough to relax. Midwives and doulas have told me that birthing people's mothers can often stop labor. Things are humming along until a mom shows up, and boom, it's like someone pressed the pause button. Nameless hospital attendants revolving in and out of the room can have a similar effect.

The second need is *quiet*. Loud sounds can cause stress and interfere with concentration. The third is physical *comfort*. Support pillows, hydration, temperature control, and movement are all labor needs, not amenities.

Physical relaxation is fourth. It's really hard to relax all of your muscles, but it's key to succumbing to contractions. *Controlled breathing* is fifth—regular and rhythmic, not panting or holding. The sixth is *closed eyes*, or the "appearance of sleep." This ensures that visual distractions don't remove the birther from planet labor.

These six labor needs permit birthers to relax. Relaxation is the key to labor. Without it, birth stalls. The needs of birthing bodies, most of all to relax, are primal and supported by decades of research and countless firsthand accounts by midwives. Not to mention by eons of women telling their own birth stories. They are prerequisites, not preferences. And yet we don't learn about them or value them as central as we prepare to give birth. Hospitals are designed to deny them all.

Ironically, and tragically, meeting these needs is associated with less pain, not more. Denying them causes more pain, which leads to more managed care, more control of birthing people.

IN GENESIS, WHEN EVE EATS FROM THE KNOWLEDGE TREE, HER descendants are punished with excruciating birth. This idea has been transmuted into our bones, morphing from religious fable into scientific fact. Generations of men have used this story to lend support to the idea that pain in labor is necessary. Pain—and possible death—as necessary punishment lay at the root of womanhood in Judaism, Islam, and Christianity.

It's no wonder that the ritual of birth has been enmeshed with superstition throughout history. For millennia, women used talismans and customs designed to help them withstand the pain and to ward off the death they heard about or witnessed. Medieval women drafted wills upon learning they were pregnant. Victorians closed doors and windows to block the bad humors, a term that came to mean bodily fluids and later moods, which were thought to bring sickness and pain. They opened drawers and cupboards and untied knots, symbolic gestures that they believed would open a woman's womb and ease labor's arduousness. Birthers wore or held charms, gemstones, amulets, magnets, coral, and jasper during their labors as totems of defense. Poor women clutched parchment or cheese inscribed with Bible verses.

Expectations of birth still hewed to Eve's punishment, though. Birth was *supposed* to hurt. If it didn't, something was wrong with the woman doing it. She wasn't morally pure or a real woman. This philosophy allowed religious men to become the supervisors of women's suffering. Men couldn't attend births, but priests could, and sometimes did, to witness labor pain. And religious leaders prohibited midwives from offering pain relief on the grounds that it threatened God's will for women. Midwives only surreptitiously offered tinctures and tools to soothe pain: eagle dung, herbs, rosewater, sugar, vinegar, and even alcohol. When Queen Victoria received chloroform during the 1853

delivery of her seventh child, Prince Leopold, the church chastised
her doctor, and he was told that "he had no right 'to rob God of the
deep, earnest cries' of women in childbirth."

In the mid-nineteenth century, doctors gave anesthesia to wounded
Civil War soldiers, but the dictate that God intended labor to be painful kept them from dispensing it to women giving birth. Men also
made judgments about whether women had suffered enough to be celebrated. "Contractions have been described by midwives, surgeons,
priests, mothers alike as 'pains,' and even as punishment. Instead of
visualizing a functional physical process the woman may perceive herself simply as invaded by pain," explains Adrienne Rich.

We still see it that way. Labor isn't power or a process; it is women's
deserved suffering validated by men's presence.

"WHATEVER YOU DO, DON'T GET PITOCIN," MY FRIEND MARGARET
said as she unsnapped the side of her bra to nurse her baby. Years before I was pregnant, we were sitting in a San Francisco kitchen that
didn't belong to us, persimmons dripping from a bowl. The owners
were winemakers renting their house to our friends, who, like us at the
time, didn't have or necessarily want children. Margaret was the only
one of us who did.

Margaret hadn't wanted to speed up a labor that the hospital believed to be too slow. After they administered the Pitocin, she said she
felt like she lost control. As if she'd been thrust down a path she hadn't
planned for and didn't want. And the pain, she said, was otherworldly.

I remember little else about her birth story—just the Pitocin, a
word I had never heard before. It is the drug meant to mimic the hormone oxytocin, integral to birth and to love. The origin of the word is
Greek, *oxys* and *tokos*, together meaning "quick birth." I was still unsure whether I would give birth myself. Whatever was to be, I decided,
I would remember this warning about Pitocin, the synthetic oxytocin.
How, as Margaret said, if I could avoid it, I could stay in control. How
it *caused* pain.

Becoming pregnant, I feared pain. I don't know how this terror became lodged in me, but I'm sure it was bound up in my knowledge of the place from which a baby was going to emerge, the vagina, an at once coveted and disparaged part. I was scared of a head passing through mine. In a children's book about childbirth that I read my kids now, the vagina is described as stretchy, to allow the baby passage, and then able to return to its previous shape. I like that image. I had heard birth breaks a person. But this kids' literature explained that expanding and contracting—resilience, really—is the vagina's job.

Margaret's was the first birth story I learned in detail. She had prepared for and expected one thing to transpire, then an entirely different thing had. I saw this as injustice, but personal to Margaret, nothing more. Still, it was fine. She was fine. The proof was her squishy baby gulping milk in a tropical shirt, charming everyone. Looking at her, my friends and I all began to yearn for something we hadn't thought to want before.

SYNTHETIC OXYTOCIN IS ONE OF THE MOST ADMINISTERED MEDIcines in labor. Doctors give it to birthing people to induce uterine contractions, to speed up labor deemed too slow, and to prompt expulsion of the placenta after the baby is born. It creates contractions that feel more intense than natural contractions, necessitating the need for pain management. Hospitals give Pitocin knowing that an epidural, numbing women below the waist, will follow.

Contractions induced by synthetic oxytocin caused many of my survey respondents tremendous pain. Eli, Bridget, and Katie called Pitocin-induced labor excruciating. Bridget wished it hadn't been given to her so soon. Medical staff gave Pitocin to JT in New Jersey without her consent. Pitocin contractions were the hardest part of labor for Ali, Alison, Victoria, Lindsay, Evan, Tori, and Rebecca. A number of women believed they were pressured or forced into Pitocin because they are Black.

The drug has existed for almost seventy years. A 2014 study found that synthetic oxytocin is administered in 57 percent of labors nationwide. Its use skyrocketed during the Covid-19 crisis as doctors ramped up their active management of the labor process, banning doulas, family members, and even partners from delivery wards and putting labor on a schedule before it began.

Synthetic oxytocin's near total adoption would suggest we understand what it is and does, its risks and benefits. But we do not. Not well enough, anyway. A primary reason for the drug's creation was to reduce cesarean births. It hasn't done that. One study found that it did the opposite: high levels of synthetic oxytocin increased risk of cesarean section.

Even dosing for the drug hasn't been standardized. More than a dozen researchers analyzed the timing and amount of synthetic oxytocin delivered to laboring women across twelve countries and in 2020 published their results in the journal *PLOS One*. They discovered that there was no established regimen for the drug—neither consistency in how often it was delivered nor a precise amount calculated in each dose, findings they called "inexplicable." The total dose infused over an eight-hour period ranged from two to twenty-seven units—a more than elevenfold difference, hinging, randomly, on where one gave birth. Other research had previously found that there is no standard dose of synthetic oxytocin. But this 2020 report was unique in that it highlighted the vast differences in drug regimens within the same country. The greatest maximum regimen and the lowest minimum regimen were both found in Germany (27 and 2.38 units, respectively). So, depending on which German hospital a pregnant person checks into, she'll get a vastly different amount of the same drug, intended for the same purpose.

"It is crucial that the appropriate minimum regimen is administered because synthetic oxytocin is a potentially harmful medication with serious consequences for women and babies when inappropriately used," explained the research team, who cautioned that we don't know what a safe amount is. They recommend studying it and hospital protocols further. Astoundingly, regulators haven't looked closely enough at the drug to intimately understand its benefits and harms. Nor have we investigated it alongside how people birth and how their babies fare.

"How can it be that we give oxytocin to almost all women in the developed world without knowing what it really does? No other drug would be given in such large amounts without being tested," said one of the paper's authors, Kerstin Uvnäs Moberg, who has studied oxytocin for more than thirty years. Moberg has found that synthetic oxytocin can make labor harder and more painful for the mother, not easier.

"We find that mothers who have had synthetic oxytocin drips can sometimes be less open ... less relaxed with higher cortisol levels," Moberg told Kathleen McCaul Moura, writing for *Granta* in 2017. "If the mother is more stressed in labour the baby gets less oxygen and less blood. In high amounts, it causes longer lasting contractions which can damage the baby," Moberg said.

No one discusses these realities at prenatal visits or the hospital bedside, where IVs are plunged into arms after extensive pressure or without permission at all. My doula told me to state my refusal firmly and to multiple nurses. "Sometimes they put it into the IV fluid without telling you," she said. "Even if you just need hydration, they'll give you oxytocin to get the placenta out faster. To move you along."

PAIN IS PROTECTIVE. IT CAN BE INSTRUCTIVE. WHEN MY ONE-year-old scalded his hand on our radiator, he removed it. The blisters that rose up, like nature's Band-Aids, helped heal him from the inside, the hospital burn specialist said. The pain ensured that he didn't immediately repeat the action, and the blisters kept him from using his hand and damaging it further while healing took place.

There are many kinds of pain. But whether we are burned, banged, or cut, the pain activates adrenaline. Next, we have a choice—fight, freeze, or escape the danger.

Is labor like burning your hand or cutting your skin? Is it an inherent distress? Is it an action that the body must protect itself against? "Feel the burn" was a phrase popularized during the onslaught of 1980s exercise videos. "No pain, no gain" is also a common adage in the diet and fitness milieu. "Just go to the point of pain, to that 'hurts so good' spot," says my exercise teacher. But I don't interpret the sensation of exercise as pain. Pain is injury. Pain means stop. "There is no physiological function in the body which gives rise to pain in the normal course of health," says Grantly Dick-Read, the British obstetrician and acclaimed author who has theorized that childbirth, a normal bodily function, is not inherently painful at all. "Against what is the uterus protecting itself by giving pain sensations in carrying out a perfectly natural function? The physiological perfection of the human body knows no greater paradox than pain in normal parturition." He blames "the young and immature" science of obstetrics for creating and reproducing the myth of labor and birth pain. A second culprit is the fear of childbirth that people are subject to from the moment they become aware of what it is and how it's done. Eve's penance. The shade thrown by religious leaders, mystics, literature, male doctors, Hollywood.

Birth isn't inherently wretched. The experience of labor, of the body's great physical and spiritual opening, doesn't have to be terrifying or unbearable. Fear of birth is a societal creation, man's projection, not a fact.

Painful isn't the word I use to describe my three natural childbirths. They were the most intense and challenging experiences of my life, some of the hardest work I have ever done. I was anxious beforehand, but in the moment I wasn't afraid. I felt seized, battered, and swallowed by the force of contractions. There were intervals during which I felt like I was being sucked into a void or knocked down by a strong surf. The sum of what I felt was intensity, hot and raw. Describing labor as pain is too simplistic. And misleading and inaccurate.

Dick-Read proposed a theory in his 1942 book *Childbirth Without Fear* to explain what causes the pain that we're not supposed to feel: the fear-tension-pain cycle. The three evils, as he calls them, are antithetical to the body's design but have been "introduced in the course of civilization by the ignorance of those concerned with preparations for an attendance at childbirth." He concludes that "the more civilized the people, the more pain of labour appears to be intensified."

The book can feel pejorative and coddling. Dick-Read believes that women's purpose is to give birth. I found this Madonna complex hard to stomach. But women weren't really Dick-Read's audience. He was speaking to his obstetric colleagues. Other men. He wanted them to stop drugging, cutting, and manipulating the birthing body when it was awesomely capable of ushering out a baby without those painful interventions. He anticipated contemporary research finding that such abuses threaten women and their bodies. He was so focused on reaching medical doctors that he even dedicated the book to Joseph DeLee, father of the "drug them and cut the baby out" school of obstetrics. It was a challenge and a plea: women *can* give birth and, in the right conditions, avoid pain.

Dick-Read developed his fear-tension-pain theory not through his course of medical study but by observing birth. "There was a calm, it seemed almost faith, in the normal and natural outcome of childbirth," he writes. The formative experience he recounts came from a casual remark a woman made to him after he attended her birth. Dick-Read rode his bicycle there in the rain. The small flat, in a poor area of London, had broken windows and a candle, lodged in a beer bottle, to light the room. His patient was naked beneath sacks and old clothes. There was no soap or towel; Dick-Read brought his own. There was "no fuss or noise," he writes. He offered her chloroform, through a face mask, when the baby's head was already crowning. Her refusal surprised him. After the baby was born, he asked her why she had declined the sedative.

"It didn't hurt. It wasn't meant to, was it, doctor?" she replied. He returns to this scene repeatedly in his text. It is his epiphany, the moment he first realizes that birth pain isn't congenital.

Dick-Read admits that it's hard to explain why one woman suffers during labor and another appears to endure it pain-free. He lands on fear as the culprit. Fear of birth pain produces the real thing. Its presence can be strong enough to alter the experience from intensity to agony. He quotes a paper in the *British Medical Journal* citing a connection between mental state and "pain originating in the pelvic viscera." He describes how fear works in the body, how it restricts the muscles, pulling them rigid and taut, like violin strings, and how this action— from fine facial muscles to toes—constricts the whole corpus:

Unfortunately the natural tension produced by fear influences those muscles which close the womb and oppose the dilation of the birth canal during labour. Therefore, fear inhibits; that is to say, gives rise to the resistance at the outlet of the womb, when in the normal state those muscles should be relaxed and free from tension. This resistance gives rise to pain, because the uterus is supplied with sensitive nerve endings which record pain arising from excessive tension.

The solution to the syndrome, Dick-Read proposes, is to "relieve tension and to overcome fear in order to eliminate pain." In other words, the work of eliminating labor pain is in the mind.

IN THE DECADES SINCE THE PUBLICATION OF DICK-READ'S BOOK, studies have provided good evidence that labor pain can be mitigated. A 2016 clinical trial of 114 women in Iran between the ages of eighteen and thirty-five aimed "to evaluate the impacts of normal physiologic childbirth on labor pain relief." Half the women were offered pregnancy and labor support designed to prevent labor pain; the other half were given conventional care. The intervention group received eight sessions of birth preparation starting at twenty weeks' gestation. During labor itself, each person was assigned an individual, reliable labor support person. The women could move freely and eat and drink during labor and birth. Once the baby arrived, they did skin-to-skin contact and breastfeeding. Those supporting labor emphasized nonpharmacological pain-relief measures—aromatherapy, heat, acupressure, music, relaxation techniques, and more. The control group did not take preparatory classes or receive individualized birth companions. They labored under complete bed rest and delivered lying on their backs. They were encouraged to push on command. Midwives attended everyone's birth.

Scientists measured the amount of pain between contractions during various stages of labor and found that women who had completed the support program reported less severe labor pain. When birthers weren't prepared, were not allowed to move around, and were instructed to push in a supine position, their births hurt more. "Fear of vaginal delivery, anxiety, tension, and unfamiliarity with the environment bring sentiments of profound insecurity for women during labor," researchers wrote in the journal *Maedica* in 2018. "It seems that there is a close connection among maternal anxiety and severity of labor pain."

This study supports what midwives and birthing people have long known: preparedness, support, freedom to move, trust in the process, and touch decrease pain. These tactics not only invite labor and birth but encourage a positive experience of it. Fear and then pain increase with the absence of these things.

RELAXING AND FEELING COMFORTABLE AND CARED FOR DURING birth reduces pain, yet hospitals operate as if this isn't known. They belittle and dismiss pain rather than work to minimize it.

Many of my survey respondents said that their labor pain wasn't managed or taken seriously by their providers. Deja in Conway, Arkansas, and Whitley in Bossier City, Louisiana, said that their doctors didn't understand or try to help when they were in pain. Courtney in Rockport, Maine, said that the triage nurse dismissed her pain because "it wasn't damaging to the baby." Some women wanted supported birth without pain medication, but their obstetricians mocked or spited them for trying.

Rebecca in Utah said she wanted a natural birth but that her doctor said "it was harder for him (his words)." He instead pressured her to be induced. Rebecca remembered that "when he broke my water, he was unnecessarily rough. It was so painful. And then "he immediately left the room and said, 'I bet you're rethinking that natural birth, aren't you?'" By then her "confidence was shot," and she was convinced that the obstetrician, as she put it, "didn't care about my comfort as a woman."

Bridget in Pennsylvania recalled being "mocked" by her obstetrician, who was a woman, "for expressing how painful" her contractions were after she was induced with Pitocin. In Chicago, Laura had "hoped to give birth without an epidural" but was induced "to speed up" her labor. She found herself "in a great deal of pain." "The male anesthesiologist, who apparently wanted to get it out of the way so he could nap, came in to pressure me into an epidural multiple times," she explained. He told her this choice would be safer if she ended up needing an emergency C-section, even though her labor was progressing normally and there was no indication for surgery. Laura tried to labor in a tub in her room, but the contractions became so intense that she agreed to the only pain relief offered—the epidural. The anesthesiologist chided, "Are you sure you don't want to try another bubble bath?"

Adriwash, in Morgantown, West Virginia, felt that her pain was dismissed because of her race. She said that her obstetrician tried to force her into an epidural and had previously tried to push her into an induction weeks earlier. The doctor was both "insensitive and verbally abusive," she said. Adriwash believes that the obstetrician, a woman, "did not take my pain seriously in the way that many practitioners working with Black patients do not."

The medical historian John Hoberman has catalogued the racist approach to labor pain tolerance that has long pervaded obstetrics. In an essay titled "The Primitive Pelvis," he explains that old "unspoken assumptions" about Black birthing bodies have been "adapted to modern circumstances," rendering them "eligible for special medical hardships." Meaning that the racist belief that Black women have higher pain tolerances and cruder birth canals than white women lives on in medical school education and practice. Racist folklore is passed on, via attitudes and anecdotes, from doctors to colleagues and students and, it appears, in the kind of care women receive. There is a direct causal relationship between these attitudes and Black people's pain and suffering during childbirth.

Anthropologist Khiara Bridges, who authored an ethnography of pregnant people seeking care in a New York City public hospital—mostly Black and Brown people on Medicaid—reveals how these tropes underly what doctors tell themselves about the care Black birthers deserve. Sometimes this occurs in code. A senior attending physician she interviewed told her that "culture" is a factor in why many patients suffer more:

I think it's cultural. Somebody coming from the middle of Africa someplace is going to have a lot more issues than somebody coming from eastern Long Island is going to have. Plus, you're going to have issues of indigency, lack of education, the whole . . . It's just poor people. Poor people don't have the same level of education obviously. They don't eat as well. They have a lot of obesity because they eat a lot of fast food and things of that nature. These are all things that are built into a clinic setting that you're not going to see elsewhere.

In this doctor's opinion, the higher rates of pathology are caused by nonwhiteness. If Black birthers are indigent, less educated, and more pain tolerant, consume poorer diets, and suffer more anyway because of their "culture" than other birthers, then providers can blame patients for complications that arise in their pregnancies or births. Perhaps they are offered less birth assistance, less supportive care. If Black women are more pain tolerant than other women, why give them pain medication if they ask for it, or why give them the needed amount if you believe they can do with less? If they're asking for too much?

When LaToya Jordan, a writer in New York City who is Black, was wheeled into surgery, she was already numb from an epidural and was promised that she wouldn't feel a thing. But when the surgeon began to make the incision for her cesarean section, she felt pain and said so. "They kept on saying, 'You feel pressure, not burning.' I was groaning and making noises, and I was really feeling it. And so, my husband is like, 'Are you OK?' 'No, I'm not OK,'" LaToya told me.

The anesthesiologist beside LaToya didn't offer to help. Finally, LaToya's husband spoke up, saying, "Can you give her something? Can you do something? She's in pain."

"Well, I can give you some more, but I don't want to give you too much because no one should be loopy or not present for your daughter's birth," the anesthesiologist told them. He administered more meds, but only after LaToya's husband asked. At the time she was relieved when the burning and pain ceased. She now feels like she was disbelieved and dismissed.

"I have a pretty high tolerance for pain," she said. "I don't know if it's people not believing women's pain is the same level as men's pain. But with Black women it's like—our pain is just not believed."

Priya, a New York lawyer and mother of two, felt searing pain in her stomach during her pregnancy, which stumped her healthcare providers. Through research, Priya learned that she was feeling the tearing of her stomach muscles as the baby grew during her first pregnancy, which is rare but real. She told her doctor what she had discovered. He didn't believe her and began treating her with suspicion. Priya is Southeast Asian and believes that because of her appearance, her doctor thought that she was trying to score painkillers. He refused to prescribe anything to alleviate her pain.

When I stumbled into triage, climbed onto all fours, and began to make sounds, like the mammal I am, I saw how the hospital workers saw me. They didn't see strength or nature. They looked afraid that I would launch a baby out of my body right there before anyone donned gloves or face shields. I wasn't in pain. I wasn't afraid. *They* were.

Because we know how we are seen in labor, it isn't a stretch to imagine that we could take on others' fear and pain and feel it ourselves. The Bradley book and Gaskin warn about this. Sociologist James McKenna describes how medical attitudes toward the birthing body interpret it as a "lethal weapon over which neither the mother nor the infant has control." Hospitals treat the birthing body as a threat, with skepticism and fear. This causes us to fear ourselves. McKenna has asked why a creator—be it Mother Earth, some ooze, or a presence in the sky—would design a mother's body as a weapon that threatens her own child. If this were reality, how would our species survive?

When pain occurs during childbirth, support structure and location can change the story. For Susanna, who gave birth at home in Long Island City, New York, the care made all the difference. Her baby was in a posterior position—that is, head down but facing forward—which caused agonizing back pain.

"I had envisioned breathing calmly through the contractions, but since the pain was more intense, I just had to sort of cope and get through them," she said. "Being under the care of midwives and others who treated this like a normal, healthy process rather than an emergency or illness really helped me stay calm and focused." Her birth story is one not of pain but of gratitude.

PAIN WAS VERY REAL TO ME THE FIRST TIME I LABORED IN THE MOments when I felt afraid. My water broke on a January morning as I was standing over a bowl of oatmeal. I had been preparing to walk to a yoga class. Instead, I ran to the bathroom to examine my drenched pants. I searched *What to Expect When You're Expecting* and then Google for when contractions should begin. Ben and I readied ourselves. The playlist! The pillows! The oil diffuser! Our plan was to labor at home for as long as possible. But then the contractions began, and how they felt changed everything.

The first few were manageable; I lay on my side resting atop cushions and relaxed into them with ease. But quickly, within minutes, they began to intensify, cramping my insides, rippling into each other. Ben tried to time them, but they didn't adhere to logic. They were already a minute apart, thirty seconds apart, so close together as to signal not labor's beginning but its end. It felt as though one would begin before the previous one ceased.

I writhed, moved into the shower, swiped bottles from the bench so I could lean against it as water pelted my back. I remember screaming. Forcefully exhaling. Thinking: They're going to have to cut this baby out of me—unsure who "they" even were. I'd been in labor for thirty minutes and had already lost hope. If this was what labor felt like at the outset, I wouldn't make it to the end. I didn't know that I was both at the beginning *and* near the end, that I was experiencing precipitous birth. My baby was practically crowning and within the hour would breathe air.

The story I told myself, the narrative I was constructing when contractions hit me like a brick wall, was that this was the beginning, there was much more ahead, and maybe I wasn't strong enough. In retrospect, I was confronting the signpost of doubt that Bradley identified as typical in labor. Before transitioning from cervix-opening contractions to the baby's emergence, women often experience hesitancy, uncertainty, and even fear of death. I didn't know what was happening. Or how long it would happen for. I was afraid.

The story we tell about how we experience pain in our bodies matters immensely, perhaps more than the fact of pain itself. This is evident in placebo research. Its progenitor, Henry Beecher, built the field studying soldiers' pain-relief measures during World War II.

When Beecher was a battlefield doctor, he was forced to ration morphine to soldiers suffering gunshot wounds. He asked them, Are you in pain? to determine who needed the medicine most. Shockingly, the majority—75 percent—said no. Beecher compared this to gunshot wound patients at his clinic in Boston before the war. He found that the "intensity of pain associated with being shot was lower in the battlefield than in civilian life," according to Daniel Carr, former president of the American Academy of Pain Medicine. Soldiers felt less pain from their gunshot wounds than civilians did. But why?

Beecher believed that the difference between two men with the same injury was context. "Meaning that the pain that you feel when you're hit by a bullet, it's not just about the bullet. It's about the story that comes with the bullet," as Robert Krulwich of Radiolab put it. For a soldier, surviving that bullet translates to heroism, awards, going home, being alive. For a civilian, it means hospital bills, lost wages and work, painful recovery without reward, quotidian concerns. One bullet, two different stories, two conflicting experiences of pain.

Whether or not we feel pain is shaped, second by second, not only by our sensory experience and by those around us but also by who we tell ourselves we are when we feel it—or when we don't. The intense pain of crowning at my labor's start wasn't the whole of my labor. It wasn't the only story. Once Sarah, our doula, arrived and was able to examine me and share what was happening, we had new information. I wasn't at labor's start; I was at labor's end. The head was right there. That changed the story that I was crafting. Sarah, seeing me labor, showed me through her tone, body language, and facial expressions that I was fine, that what I was experiencing was natural, typical even, and that eased my fear. I could do this if I was safe and it wouldn't be for much longer.

Could we make it to the hospital? We decided to try, as I didn't want an ambulance ride with an infant after an unplanned home birth, an occurrence that would surely ensue if I stayed put and called 911. We piled into an Uber, me in slippers, pajamas, and a T-shirt I had slept in the night before, beneath my winter coat from the Costco men's department. Ben and Sarah briefed the driver on the seriousness of our mission. I knelt on the floor of the backseat of his car, breathing two short breaths out and one in, literally sucking the baby back inside, as Sarah coached me. The story changed. Now I wasn't a sufferer withstanding a bodily assault, but a warrior pursuing a goal, hurtling to the place where I planned to give birth. I needed to not give birth in this car crossing the Gowanus Canal.

Bless you, the driver repeated. Bless you.

His words swelled my heart, constructed a story of my worthiness and even heroism as we moved forward, my face resting on the cool tang of black leather, knees grinding into the dirty floor. In the car, I didn't feel pain. I didn't feel pain walking slowly to the elevator, which Ben commandeered. Nor did I feel it on all fours on a gurney in triage. Intensity, yes, like waves breaking into walls. Gripping like a fist. But pain? No.

CHAPTER 4
CHILDBEARING HIPS

WHEN I WAS IN HIGH SCHOOL, I WASTED TIME PASSING NOTES
with two boys whose minds I wanted but not their bodies or
faces. I think they felt the reverse about me. We sat in wooden desks in
a classroom attached to the chemistry lab. There was a life-size model
skeleton on wheels, lines of tables, beakers. It smelled like the formal-
dehyde used to preserve dissection specimens—frogs, fetal pigs, and,
most recently, cats. We filleted actual house pets in there, hindquar-
ters so large that they looked like a different species. I wouldn't touch
them and gagged when we discovered one had been expecting.

In the notes, I wrote about the kind of music we liked or didn't, up-
coming sporting events or social gatherings. The boys sent sketches
of penises, or comic violence, or sometimes bodies that looked like
mine. These exchanges made the minutes pass. One day, the teacher
snatched the note. I hadn't thought her the type until she did it, oblong
nails impaling the lined paper, glasses shielding her brow as she read.

Back there, she said, pointing to the last row. I stood, turned, and grabbed my things. With those childbearing hips of yours, she added.

I felt my chest tear. I slunk to the punishment desk, dodging stares, desperate to know what she meant. I hated that she had drawn attention to a part of my body that I already worried about. The hips that, in store dressing rooms, I squeezed into the kind of pants my mother wouldn't let me buy.

I had thought about my hips critically, about the way they could fill certain clothes in an unattractive way, the shame of them bare at the pool, but not about what they might be capable of, what they could produce or endure. I was ashamed of the reproductive role the teacher had assigned me. To call my body "childbearing" was to say that I was capable of it, that I knew how to get a baby in there. She, a female adult, was sexualizing me in front of a group of kids, my peers, in a way that was both overt and confounding. That it had come from a woman, rather than a man, took me by surprise, maybe making it worse.

I had written chemistry formulas upside down on my stomach ahead of a test in her class. Sagged my flesh so my tight top would snap up like a roller shade and reveal the answers, which I then copied down. Maybe she had seen me.

She also drew a line from motherhood to me, a teenage girl. What business did I have with mothers? Those people drove Suburbans and got divorced. The teacher was much older than me, already a mother, but she had typically treated me with a warmth I had, until that moment, enjoyed. Maybe she leapt over that line because she liked me. The remark had been delivered with something like a smile. Or maybe, in some strange, unintentional way, she was opening a door to me, to my future. She taught science. Were hips that appeared ready to bear children good?

Hips hold tension. From sitting, walking, standing up. They absorb the shock of feet springing from the floor. They support the body's movements. They tilt and sway and pop, for sex, long sprints, to "Apache" by the Sugarhill Gang. The pelvic bowl is wide and sculptural, like jaws, encasing the life-giving organs.

My teacher humiliated me in front of my peers. Her comment was a snipe, not an actual prediction. But she happened to guess right. My body, I, we, birth extraordinarily well. If I were a character in Lois Lowry's *The Giver*, I would have lived in the birth factory, pumped full of babies. I would not have stopped at the required number; I would have owned the place. My teacher had said that I might be good at something common yet taboo. It's a radical thing to claim, to own, to take pride in. But when it comes to birth, my pelvic bones and the surrounding flesh that overfills skinny pants get it done.

I'm not the only one. Our society is steeped in narratives of dangerous and life-threatening birth, heroic doctors, and the flawed frailty of the female body. It needs more stories that acknowledge the truth: we were born to birth.

CONTEMPORARY ANTHROPOLOGY PROPOSES A COMPELLING THEory about how women's bodies evolved to give birth and why they experience it as dangerous and painful. This theory centers on the pelvis, the bony bowl at the base of the spine. Our legs, trunks, and muscles attach to it. Inside are the bladder and sex organs, tipped to the front, like an offered dish of fruit. The anthropologists tell us that women evolved wider ones than men, some three to four million years ago, so that we could birth our species' increasingly large-brained babies. They also tell us that men's narrower pelvises produce a better gait, making them faster runners than women. Women's wider pelvises, a prerequisite for ejecting infants, rendered them slower and less efficient movers than men.

The theory of the pelvic compromise between narrow (for motility) and wide (for birthing big-brained, intelligent life) creates the hostile condition of the human birth canal, which fits far more snugly around a human baby than the birth canals of other closely related primates. Human babies, then, are more taxed when exiting their mothers than orangutan, chimpanzee, and gorilla young. Childbirth is therefore more dangerous for humans and this is why we require labor assistance from other members of our species when our hairier close evolutionary cousins don't.

The second part of the pelvic compromise theory is that human babies vacate bellies earlier in their development than other primate babies—any later and their heads would be too large to traverse the birth canal. So human babies are born helpless, in need of our care. Unlike horses, giraffes, and deer, which can walk immediately after birth, human babies are floppy and useless. More creature than child. A screaming meatloaf. To be born developmentally ready to get around on their own, babies would need to gestate quite a bit longer. A good estimate is an extra seven months.

The price of bigger brains and thus higher intelligence, greater consciousness, better mobility, and much more tool use, then, appears to be strenuous, painful, potentially life-threatening childbirth. Or, as Holly Dunsworth, an associate professor of anthropology at the University of Rhode Island, put it to me, "Thanks a lot, evolution. Childbirth sucks."

THE THEORY LEAPT FROM SCIENCE TO CULTURE THROUGH THE EFforts of men. Enter Sherwood Washburn, a preeminent midcentury anthropologist and primatologist whose lectures produced standing ovations. He explained not only how we derive movement and behaviors from our ape cousins but also where we diverge. Washburn's greatest contribution to his field is a theory called the *obstetrical dilemma*—or the more formal explanation of why childbirth sucks. The idea had been kicking around insular academia, but it hadn't punctured the mainstream until 1960, when Washburn described it in *Scientific American*:

> Humans are born underdeveloped. We are born early in order to escape just in time before we outgrow the birth canal. This early birth is caused by antagonistic natural selection. While our brains got bigger and bigger over time, the evolution of bipedalism prevented our birth canals from expanding, too. Difficult, dangerous childbirth of underdeveloped, helpless human babies are both evidence of, and solutions to, this obstetrical dilemma.

Because Washburn's framing of the obstetrical dilemma appeared in a popular magazine rather than an academic journal, the idea reached a large audience. The article would extend the obstetrical dilemma's influence farther beyond Washburn's field of human evolution than he or his contemporaries could have imagined. The obstetrical dilemma has animated anthropology for more than half a century, and it's foundational to our culture of birth today. However, the idea is far better known than its name or its creator. Notably, the framework Washburn is famous for isn't mentioned in his obituary (he died in 2000) or, as of this writing, on his Wikipedia page.

It *is* a sexy idea. The bind that childbirth must be difficult and dangerous because of fixed pelvic size to optimize movement is powerful enough to "convert creationists," according to a colleague Dunsworth studied with. The colleague said that when he teaches it to students, he sees lightbulbs glowing above their heads. This is why it is taught in college science departments in classes on evolutionary biology, anthropology, anatomy, and physiology. It appears in medical school texts and undergraduate lectures alike.

Dunsworth has blonde hair and a deep dimple in her cheek when she smiles, which she often does when posing with various bones—mandibles, skulls, pelvises. She too possessed one such lightbulb. She encountered the framework as an undergraduate in the 1990s and has loved it ever since ("And who didn't?"). Dunsworth believed the obstetrical dilemma, elegant and satisfying, was "a relief because difficult childbirth and helpless infants are not Eve's fault, but rather evolution's."

The pull of the dilemma has reached beyond college curricula. My first exposure to it was through popular musician Father John Misty, a performer known for both elliptical hips and cynicism. He sings about the dilemma in the first lines of the opening song on what is, arguably, his most popular record: "Our brains are way too big for our mother's hips. So, nature, she devised this alternative. We emerge half-formed and hope whoever greets us on the other end is kind enough to fill us in."

These lyrics open "Pure Comedy," the title track of his Grammy-nominated album. They, along with his captivating performance of them at Brooklyn's Kings Theater in May 2017, attacked me like an itch. I listened to the song repeatedly. I thought about my hips and those of Josh Tillman (the man behind the Misty) and wondered if he was blaming the birth canal for humanity's fundamental inadequacies. The song's popularity ensured that women's flawed hips were everywhere, accepted. He trilled about them while gyrating on *Saturday Night Live*. The lyrics dribbled into the suburban grocery where I bought coffee filters. The verse is actually how I found Holly Dunsworth. She mentions it in a 2018 paper she wrote about the obstetrical dilemma, to establish how well known the dilemma is.

The success of influencer pediatrician Harvey Karp further proves the obstetrical dilemma's assimilation into popular culture. The foundation of Karp's theory is that newborns benefit from shushing, swaying, and sucking—throwback behaviors to their womb stay—because they were expelled early. For the first six months of life, Karp recommends treating babies like fetuses to calm them when they fuss and to encourage them to sleep. His book, *The Happiest Baby on the Block*, has sold more than a million copies and is routinely a top parenting seller on Amazon. Dog-eared paperbacks are traded in parent-dense neighborhoods and litter used bookstores nationwide. New parents describe it with a religious fervor and pass the book to one another, murmuring, "This will change your life." A neighbor gave me her paperback after my first child was born. I used it as permission to pop a pacifier in my daughter's mouth and wear her in a carrier all day and immediately regretted the few months I'd spent parenting without it.

Treating babies as if they were born early has sprouted an empire. Karp raised $30 million in investment capital to create a motorized bassinet that claims to solve for the dilemma of early birth by shushing and shuttling your baby back and forth, like a carnival ride. We rented it, and it was both incredible and horrifying—it sounds like a vacuum and is controlled with an app. But baby slept, meaning we slept. If the white noise was turned way up, I could hardly hear any cries. Sometimes I wonder whether Karp would be so popular if proper human support after childbirth were routine.

"OBSTETRICAL DILEMMA THINKING IS EVERYWHERE, AND I helped with that," Dunsworth admitted. She taught it to her students while in graduate school at Penn State and even enshrined it in a reference guide she wrote and published in 2007. For Dunsworth, who grew up in Central Florida, learning *anything* about evolution was radical, since all she heard as a kid was how evil it was. The obstetrical dilemma was more needed proof that evolution, not creation, was responsible for all of this.

Dunsworth finished her dissertation on fossil ape feet, then began to research how ape babies moved differently than their parents. She was readying herself for a journey into proving the obstetrical dilemma. Now she would have the time and freedom to track down the evidence. She didn't doubt it was there. She could hardly wait.

Dunsworth thought she would find that humans experienced shorter pregnancies than other primates. "If you know maternal body size you can predict pregnancy length," she said. "This is true across placental mammals. If you know other variables, like how big the mother's brain is and how big the baby's brain is, you can get even better results in your predictions." When Dunsworth did those calculations, she quickly learned that human pregnancies weren't shorter than those of other primates. Women don't give birth early. They give birth more or less when they're supposed to.

She began to consider the pelvic compromise that supposedly bound women and birth—stuck between narrow for good walking or running and wide enough for birthing large brains. It reminded her of an early encounter with a coach, a story that she shared with me. Dunsworth was a ten-year-old star athlete, better than her peers. Her school only had a boys' soccer team, so she asked to play on it. The coach told her no, because "I could get hurt and never be able to have babies," she recalled. "I didn't believe it. I just believed something was wrong with him. And then I realized that it's the culture." Competitive organized sports for men took off in the US much earlier than for women and still claim more money and fans. This is not because men are inherently superior at sports. It's rooted in the dogma that birthing hips can't run, kick, leap, jump, turn, dive, and push off the side of a pool as well as nonbirthing hips. This tenet is weaponized against women from the time they are children, undermining them on ballfields and elsewhere.

Anna Warrener, a Harvard anthropology professor and mom of three, also knew that women could walk and run just fine, but she wanted to prove it. The obstetrical dilemma holds that women's birth-compromised pelvises make them eternally slower, less efficient movers than men, so Warrener put both men and women on treadmills to compare. She measured stride length and the sway in their gaits. Two people who have the same pelvic dimensions can still move differently, with varying levels of efficiency, because of sway and stride length as well as the 3D dynamics of gait. Additionally, many factors influence the symphony of movement. Beyond the bones there are oxygen flow, leg length, muscle tone, height, and weight. There are conditions, such as weather, clothes, and terrain.

Warrener and her colleagues found that the evidence for Washburn's theory is lacking: "The obstetrical dilemma trade-off hypothesis that a wider pelvis is required to permit the birth of large-brained infants, but a narrow pelvis increases locomotor efficiency does not accurately represent dynamic hip abductor mechanics during locomotion." The results shouldn't have been a surprise. Men and women can both move well; women aren't worse off because of their birth canals.

Humans don't in fact experience shorter pregnancies than other species. The average woman walks and runs just as successfully as the average man. These were the ironclad supports for the obstetrical dilemma, yet they are full of holes. Dunsworth began to think about bones and about how evolutionary biologists prize them because they are easy to find and study. But bones don't tell the whole story. Metabolism, hormones, tissues, the brain, respiratory function, and more all dramatically influence birth. Yet they are far more complex and tougher to locate and study than bones. You can't hold a hormone in your hand.

The obstetrical dilemma is lore that has permeated the culture and remained, mostly, unchallenged. Reviews quoted the Father John Misty lyric but then skipped forward to his indictment of capitalism and his reference to bedding Taylor Swift in the Oculus Rift. The hip myth stands as fact. Karp's methods persuade new parents desperate to try anything in exchange for a few more minutes of sleep, and while he may help parents calm their newborns, his womb re-creation strategies "don't have a bipedal leg to stand on," Dunsworth said.

For the better part of the past decade, Dunsworth has been working to unravel the obstetrical dilemma. She gives lectures, publishes papers, conducts studies, and teaches classes. She and colleagues are impeaching the myths of primitive and defective hips and early birth of unfinished infants. The trial is ongoing. Her work has champions but also dissenters: the anthropology old guard, those who study pelvic anatomy, paleontologists with fancy titles. In other words, mostly men.

Dunsworth knew that she couldn't reject the obstetrical dilemma without offering an alternative theory. It's called energetics of gestation and growth (EGG). EGG is not about the relationship between pelvises and brain size. Pregnancy is incredibly taxing on a body's metabolism. As a baby grows, so does her mother's energy needs. Pregnant bodies are pushed to their limit, metabolically speaking. And by pregnancy's end, a baby's energy needs will inevitably surpass her mother's ability to meet them, creating a stress response—the release of hormones that may start labor. Energy needs, not brain size, prompt birth. Dunsworth says that EGG applies across mammal populations. Babies take and take from moms, and when moms can't give anymore, the babies evacuate.

Once when she gave a lecture explaining EGG, a prominent male paleontologist approached her afterward to tell her, "Nice talk. But it's not evolution."

Within the ideology that women's pelvises are subpar, there are further rankings. Early twentieth-century doctors argued that Black women were endowed with a "primitive pelvis," distinct from white women's "civilized" hips. Medical historian John Hoberman explains, in his essay "The Primitive Pelvis," how this racialized folklore created a binary mindset that crept into medical literature:

"primitive" described Black, African, African American, and Indigenous women; "civilized" mostly referred to white women of European descent. Black women were believed to be "endowed with a biological toughness and resiliency that constitute an enduring racial trait," he wrote. Their "hardiness and supernormal vitality" contrasted with white women's perceived sensitivity and weakness, leading to less support for Black women and, as I'll discuss later, more violence.

"The negro pelvis shows a reversion toward the type found in the lower animals," wrote an American physician in 1925. "The pelvis of the Negro mother is narrower and deeper than that of the white," claimed a 1932 article from the journal *Human Biology*. "Contracted pelves are about four times as frequent in Negros as in white mothers ... and are said to be common among primitive peoples in their native abodes."

But suppositions of primitiveness didn't stop there. They extended from small, underdeveloped, animalistic Black pelvises to the notion of Black babies having smaller, softer heads, better able to shimmy through a narrow birth canal. And the primitive pelvis hypothesis was used to claim that Black women had less difficult labors than white women. Researchers said that Black women were more likely to deliver spontaneously than white women, that they less often required surgery, and that their labors were shorter. Essentially, they were thought to be better at physiologic birth.

As birth became increasingly medicalized, the surgical techniques and tools forcibly developed on Black bodies were deployed to treat white ones. Doctors believed white women's bodies were weak and needy, thus deserving of medicine's best practices. Black women's bodies had been deemed "hardy"—more pain tolerant, disease resistant, and "animalistic," with a pelvic shape better adapted to birth. Physicians concluded that Black women therefore did not require—or deserve— expensive birth technology. First they were test subjects; then they were denied the very tools and procedures their bodies helped create.

Pelvises and baby heads come in different shapes and sizes. Labor and women's interpretations of its length and difficulty vary tremendously too. None of this is determined by racial characteristics alone.

Sharing a country of origin or skin color does not produce homoge-nous hips, let alone birthing experiences. These anachronistic, racist ideas belong firmly in the past. However, like the obstetrical dilemma, they inform how we view birth—and give birth—today.

THE MYTH OF THE FLAWED PELVIS SCAFFOLDS THE MODERN BIRTH industry. It perpetuates the idea that "women and their babies are fun-damentally in opposition to each other" and that "the female body is dangerous by design," birth educator and activist Cristen Pascucci told the *Washington Post* in 2016. The paper was reporting on doctors who wanted to induce everyone at thirty-nine weeks' gestation. Pas-cucci said this inclination is rooted in a mom-versus-baby mentality that "reinforces a century-old pre-feminist American obstetric view that birth is pathological, and the doctor's job is to extract the fetus from the incubator." Obstetrical dilemma thinking also fuels the no-tion that doctors rescue babies from birth. It not only excuses unnec-essary interventions in childbirth, it demands them. It is the backbone of present-day meddling with tools.

The 1960s, when Washburn published his obstetrical dilemma arti-cle, were a boom time for tool use in childbirth. Obstetric ultrasound emerged—that is, using sound waves to gauge fetal growth. Elec-tronic fetal monitoring arrived, allowing doctors to track the heart rates of mothers and babies during birth. Pelvic X-rays were still being performed on pregnant women despite their danger. When the epi-demiologist Alice Stewart identified the radiation from these X-rays as a cause of cancer in babies, her male colleagues scoffed at her conclu-sions and denied her research funding, even as more babies died. The emergence of all of this new technology in the second half of the twen-tieth century marked the moment when "attention shifted from the mother to the fetus," according to an obstetrics history in the *British Medical Journal*. Doctors began to use these interventions to obsess over babies' sizes and make conjectures about whether they would fit through the birth canal. The more doctors used technology to pry into wombs, the more their popularity spiked.

No one ever came after me threatening C-section, but that didn't mean the obstetrical dilemma was absent from how I experienced birth. When I was pregnant with my second child, my providers treated me differently at prenatal visits than they had during my first pregnancy. A lot of skimming over stuff, and comments like "You know this already" and "You've done this before." Which was true, but after some querying, I came to understand that my "proven pelvis" might have something to do with the more laissez-faire approach for round two. My obstetrician said my pelvis was more "capable," and therefore my birth might be safer than that of an unproven first-time mom. I was at less risk for all kinds of pregnancy problems. They were more at ease with me than with someone whose pelvis might be "incapable." Neophyte birthers were like LOL Surprise dolls—when you got the package, you didn't know what was inside. Professional birth people describing my pelvis as "proven" made me feel confident and good. Like my body was somehow protected by previous experience. I did wonder whether I felt safer because they had told me my birth should be easier or because their belief in my easier second birth meant that they wouldn't mess with me.

Obviously, moms can be more prepared for their second births. But the opposite of proven isn't novice; it's untested, false. First-time birthers shouldn't be invalidated or deemed complicated before they even try. My second birth took four times as long as my first one. Both were wonderfully uncomplicated. It didn't matter whether my pelvis was "proven" or not. The term only grafted someone else's beliefs and expectations onto me. And doesn't "proven pelvis" sound an awful lot like "primitive pelvis," a term that serves no one? I wonder why it's necessary to label pelvises at all. Categorizing them doesn't appear to better birth experiences or outcomes.

If the obstetrical dilemma is flawed and its application misogynistic and racist, why does it remain influential? Once a finding catches fire, it can be tough to extinguish. The reasons are practical and political. Washburn was a pioneer in the field of human evolution. He and his contemporaries and those who came after them, who knew and sowed this idea, were men. Younger or less successful scientists resist challenging the ideas of accomplished figures. Even if they too are white men, as was the case for human evolutionary biology in the 1950s and 1960s.

"It was mostly men doing this work who weren't bearing children," Dunsworth observed. It can often take an outsider to see an idea from a different angle to question and dispute its veracity. Dunsworth is a scientist with tenure. She's also a woman. And unlike Washburn and his male colleagues, who privileged bones, she has given birth. And she did so, to her dismay, with the full arsenal of modern drugs and tools.

"They pointed at the calendar and said, 'Well, we're all going to jail if we don't induce by this date, so pick a night when your favorite midwife is on and we will schedule your induction,'" Dunsworth recalled, with a dark laugh. She didn't want an induction, and it wasn't clear that she needed one. The provider's appeal to jailtime was less a real possibility than a threat.

"I'm super into knowing things and investigating things and I try to be a good scholar and scientist," she said. But when facing induction, she was afraid to ask questions. "As soon as I knew we were going to induce, I knew that my chances for a C-section had gone way up." She was suspected of having a big baby: "Fire fighters would lean out of their trucks and shout, 'Are you OK?' when I was just walking down the street. I was huge."

At first, all was well. Dunsworth napped to conserve energy, a normal, useful tactic, but one her doctors rejected. "They're like no, no, no. And then they just ramped it up to hell. They burst my bag. I was on all the drugs. I was vomiting between contractions. It was a botched induction. And then they said, 'You could keep going like this for twenty hours and end up with a C-section or have a C-section now.' I got a C-section because they wouldn't give me time, and I'm never going to forgive them. I'm so angry still. It's been almost five years."

Dunsworth's baby was healthy, large, and nursed with ease. Her experience giving birth and her lens on the subject makes her that crucial "other" in her field. She can challenge what has supposedly been settled.

WHAT HAS BEEN PERCEIVED AS A UNIQUELY FEMALE FLAW ISN'T A flaw at all.

"One might say that women's hips are *more* adapted than men's, given natural selection did not just build them as cornerstones of bipedalism but also as gateways for the ever-evolving species," Dunsworth told me. "Women's bodies are highly adapted for complex functionality, and they are not 'compromised' unless the narrator is stuck in obstetrical dilemma thinking."

Oh, how we are stuck.

"It's been a story that everyone who has any sort of formal academic experience in human evolution, or human anatomy, has been exposed to," Dunsworth said. "If you've been exposed to these ideas, if you're in a delivery room, including if you're the mother in labor, then it's going to affect you. It's going to help you give up earlier. It's going to help you give into what you think is evolved human nature and just use another form of evolved human nature—tools!—to intervene instead. I know this knowledge has contributed to the rise of medical intervention in childbirth."

Modern obstetrics still preaches that birth is a battle between mother and child and worries that babies grow too large to safely exit the bodies that built them. However, obstetricians cannot accurately discern a baby's size in utero toward the end of a pregnancy, according to recent studies. When ultrasounds predict big babies, they are wrong about half the time, far too frequently to be relied upon. This fact has not stopped doctors from inducing or scheduling surgery for pregnant people, essentially claiming they cannot birth their own babies, that their babies won't fit through the birth canal before they have even tried. Despite obstetric alarm sounding, what we know hardly suggests that women routinely build babies too large to birth.

That obstetricians cannot accurately discern a baby's size in utero has not stopped their meddling. About one in three women is told she will have a big baby at the end of pregnancy when only one in ten does. Actually, birthing a larger-than-average baby is far less risky to a pregnant person than her doctor thinking she is carrying one. One study compared women whose doctors suspected they were carrying large babies (babies bigger than eight pounds, thirteen ounces) with women who gave birth to large babies that doctors hadn't anticipated. The group predicted to have big babies was three times more likely to be induced, more than three times as likely to have C-sections, and four times as likely to have birth complications. Far more problematic than a big baby is the need to intervene.

THE EVIDENCE FOR WHY THE PELVIS IS ACTUALLY SUPREMELY evolved for birthing large-brained babies is the millennia humans have spent successfully doing just that. Yes, it *is* a tighter fit between head and bones than in nonhuman primates or even earlier human-like species. But both birthing and baby bodies have adapted in astounding ways.

Some of them are physical. "Both the fetal skull and the birthing pelvis are able to change shape significantly to accommodate each other," says Megan Davidson, a doula who has attended more than seven hundred births. Davidson, author of a book called *Your Birth Plan*, emphasizes that the modern pelvis isn't a door baby enters; rather, the baby moves through it with a series of rotations. In digital animations of the journey, the baby appears to be spinning, doing cartwheels and somersaults.

In addition to performing distinct choreography, baby's body shapeshifts to get out. "Their skull bones can move closer together or even overlap to mold their head so that it can travel through the pelvis," Davidson told me. Squishy, stretchy babies adapted big brains but also soft, mobile heads to fit through their mothers' birth canals. Mom's hormones encourage pliability in the ligaments that hold her bones together—pelvises widen during the fertile years and, of course, during pregnancy and birth. In one animation I saw, the pelvic bones appear to swing open like double doors. These adaptations seem to disprove the argument that birthing pelvises are the wrong shape and size to birth, that they lack compatibility with their babies. Labor is like two bodies dancing, not fighting.

Pelvises aren't proportioned the same. Anthropologists Lia Betti and Andrea Manica measured 348 skeletons from around the world and found enormous variation in size and shape. "The significant extent of canal shape variation among women from different regions of the world has important implications for modern obstetric practice in multi-ethnic societies, as modern medical understanding has been largely developed on studies of European women," the researchers wrote in 2018.

Betti and Manica found that pelvic shape correlated to geography. People from sub-Saharan Africa had the deepest pelvises, Native Americans had the widest. Europeans, North Africans, and Asians weren't quite as deep or wide. These findings suggest that race and geography play a role in pelvic shape, not that they determine it.

Still, modern doctors may center one type of pelvis. "What worries me is that doctors come out of school thinking of the European model of the pelvis," Betti told the *New York Times* in 2018. The belief among obstetricians that only one type of pelvis is "normal" has led to unnecessary interventions like induction, forceps use, and cesarean section, "which can further exacerbate harm." For instance, views that all pelvises are the same, like those of Europeans, have encouraged violence performed on nonwhite women. Betti gave an example of a doctor using forceps on a Black woman to try to rotate her baby to traverse a white, European pelvic shape, the one he understood. Anatomy professor Helen Kurki told the *New York Times* that these findings challenge the thinking that "there is one 'right' way to birth a baby." They also indicate that Black women are oppressed by both myth and fact. Doctors make discriminatory medical decisions about them based on racist myths while simultaneously ignoring actual biological differences across racial groups.

Ultimately, why we birth the way we do transcends the boundaries of our bones. Physiologic labor is a complex process involving, yes, bones, but also tissues, muscles, organs, cells, hormones, an exchange of signals between two people, mechanical changes, emotions. Bones are easier to see and study, so bone shape and size are what obstetricians, historians, and anthropologists have historically prioritized.

Some anthropologists believe the tight fit, the mom-baby birth canal dance, and the fact that babies emerge facing *away* from their mothers are proof that we evolved to *require* birth support. That birthing alone isn't just undesirable, it's not what we're meant to do.

The constraints of the evolutionary process have "resulted in heightened emotional needs during labour, which lead women to seek companionship at this time," wrote anthropologists Karen Rosenberg and Wanda Trevathan in their paper "Birth, Obstetrics, and Human Evolution," published in 2002. "To put it in evolutionary terms, as bipedalism evolved, natural selection favoured the behavior of seeking assistance during birth," they explain. They say it wasn't a conscious call by moms; rather, it was likely driven by the brain—"fear, anxiety, pain, or desire to conform to behavioral norms." Support not only improved mortality for all involved but has become women's evolutionary birthright. They conclude that the very emotions of birth are "adaptations to the obstetric complications of bipedalism."

But the support we've evolved to seek and need has, in the hands of the American labor and delivery system, morphed into control. When hospital systems believe they know what a body is capable of better than the person whose body it is, we have a problem. Thanks to the obstetrical dilemma myth, the primitive pelvis theory, and a hyperfocus on bones, birth assistance has been bastardized. Support has devolved into manipulation on the premise that birthers' bodies are flawed. Today, knowledgeable people don't support birth so much as men govern it.

CHAPTER 5
IT'S BETTER TO BE CUT

"IT'S BETTER TO BE CUT," MY MOTHER SAYS, RUNNING HER KNIFE through a bouquet of scallions. Green ribbons scatter.

"It's true," my aunt agrees from the floor, where she snuggles a dog. "I had one."

"I had one," my mom says, abrading the frying pan with a wooden spoon.

"They have to make room for the baby to come out," my aunt says. "You're teeny," she adds, looking at my mom.

"But you stretch?" I say.

"It's so you don't tear," my aunt clarifies. The small dog has flipped over to enjoy a belly rub. "That's a good boy."

"You can still tear if you get cut. You can tear more," I say, thinking back to birth class. But I can't remember exactly.

They look at each other for a long moment.

"I went to sleep, and when I woke up, I was a mom," says my

grandmother from her bar stool. She is wearing sunglasses indoors.

"They cut you too," my aunt tells her. My grandmother shrugs. Her eyebrows jump above the frames.

"I didn't feel a thing."

"It's easier to stitch a straight line than a tear," my mom says. "The straight line heals better." She's been to the fridge, the oven, and the pantry. She hovers now over a sink full of celery.

"It's better than tearing," says my aunt.

"That's not true," I say, my voice rising. "I don't think that's true."

"Yes, it is," my mom says, a little louder.

"I tore, and I healed just fine," I say, not knowing whether this is entirely true.

"You wanted to do it yourself," my grandmother explains.

"Not sure I had a choice," I say. "What if you weren't going to tear and they cut you anyway?"

"Everyone has one," my aunt says, snuggling the dog.

WOMEN IN MY FAMILY AND YOURS HAVE UNDERGONE EPISIOTO-mies in part because of the common fear of tearing during childbirth. For generations, we have been told that men ripping us open is preferable to what our own bodies might do.

My mom doesn't remember whether anyone told her. She hadn't had any anesthesia. No epidural. My aunt also can't remember whether or not she was told. My grandmother gave birth knocked out at what was then called Beth Israel Hospital in the East Village. She wasn't unique; her contemporaries, who gave birth in the 1950s, largely did so comatose. You can't push out a baby—or even really attend a birth—that you're not awake for. Even if it's your own.

An episiotomy is "a surgical cut made at the opening of the vagina during childbirth, to aid a difficult delivery and prevent rupture of tissues," says the *Oxford English Dictionary*. Presented this way, episiotomy sounds like a helpmate, an aid. However, the assist comes from doing exactly what the practice claims it's trying to prevent. It hinders a possible (but by no means guaranteed) rupturing of tissues by rupturing tissues. Dana Gossett, chair of obstetrics and gynecology at the University of California, likened episiotomy to tearing a shirt hem. "It's nearly impossible to rip a shirt," she told the *New York Times*, "but if I make a little nick in the hem … you'll be able to rip it all the way open."

During my first pregnancy, I feared tearing during childbirth most. I did so palpably without knowing which part of me would. The name of the anatomy was a mystery. Was it the vulva? Vagina? Clitoris? Something else? Would a tear mimic paper or fabric—a booklet, a seam, a dollar bill? I thought about what could cause a breech. Surely the descent of a mammoth cranium. Maybe another infant part, a hand or elbow, plummeting with the skull? A tear in such a delicate place would surely be torture and make sex hurt.

A natural tear or episiotomy incision typically lacerates the perineum. Growing up on women's magazines in the late 1990s, I had believed that only men had perinea. The landing strip between scrotum and anus was the title character in advice columns about man-pleasing. They were lousy with nerve endings, enjoying sensations like being licked, tickled, or stroked with ice. They were a pleasure mecca, a runway, a place to levitate from.

Women have perinea too. Unlike the gilded male desire hub, though, they have been described as flat surfaces with little purpose— or possibly, if you weren't careful, an odor. They were a place of shame. Better unnamed, concealed.

"The area between the vulva and the anus" is a textbook description of the perineum. But anatomically, the perineum is far more than a void between those borders. Its diamond-shaped structure supports key body systems. It contains a bounty: nerves, tissues, fascia, tendons, muscles, and glands. It holds both the urogenital triangle and the anal triangle, making it integral to elimination, intercourse, and childbirth. The urogenital triangle contains strong deep muscles as well as the urethra, the vagina, the clitoris, and a continuation of the abdominal muscles. The anal triangle comprises the anal sphincter and the muscles responsible for its movement. It is also a footpath for pleasure, as it houses the pudendal nerve, which carries sensation to the clitoris. I once heard a fitness instructor describe the region of the body including the perineum as the place "where all of your goodness is."

The perineum is a treasure, filled with flexibility, purpose, and brawn. It is built to stretch in childbirth. Its center point, the perineal body, contains thick, springy muscles designed to give and lengthen as an infant's head crowns. One explanation I read called the perineum a "tear-resistant body." It is designed to give, not to cleave.

WHEN I ASKED ONE OF MY MIDWIVES WHAT CAUSED TEARING AND how I could prevent it, she shrugged.

Some people tear, and some people don't, she said.

Her vagueness grated. I told myself that I would be a person who didn't. In the absence of her support, deciding that it wouldn't happen to me would be my first act of defense.

I read about tearing, anatomy, and risk, my fear being alternately stoked and dampened on a loop. Tears are fairly common—between half and three-quarters of people experience a tear or laceration during vaginal birth. Most first-degree tears involve the skin around the vaginal opening. Many birth workers say they don't require repair and heal on their own. Second-degree tears sever the perineum and require stitches. Third- and fourth-degree tears can reach the anus and rectum, respectively. They occur in 3 to 7 percent of births, but researchers suggest that with a skilled, properly trained practitioner, they can be reduced to 1 percent.

I learned that birthers who experienced tearing often didn't feel it happening. They were frozen below the waist with epidurals, or their perinea were naturally numb from birth hormones. I wasn't sure if that was more terrifying or a relief.

An informal poll found that close to 90 percent of people fear tearing in childbirth. Women have admitted to me that fear of tearing is why they decided against having kids. These fears are not necessarily misplaced. In the United States, hospitals do not publicly report the rates at which tears occur. It's practically impossible to know whether a provider's clients tear at every birth or not at all.

Recording and reporting rates are "not prioritized or considered important, which is really sad," said Rebecca Dekker, founder of Evidence Based Birth, in a webinar presenting the evidence on tear prevention. Tears aren't valued enough to document—even though they universally cause terror, pain, and harm. I also realized through my reading that prevention measures were available.

I tried to forestall tearing with Kegels, squats, a profusion of prenatal yoga. A pelvic floor physical therapist recommended perineal massage, which is less relaxing than preparatory stretching. She explained how it worked: Insert thumb into the vagina. Apply light pressure. Scoop in a U-shape along the lower rim. Regular efforts are meant to stretch the perineal muscles in advance of birth. Pro tips include loosening first in a warm bath, keeping nails short, and using a lubricant. She did the exercise to me as I lay on her table. When I tried it myself at home, it hurt, and I bled. I didn't try it again.

I read about a balloon you could inflate and insert to achieve vaginal pliability. This "birth trainer" device was both intriguing and suspect. A couple hundred dollars to preserve the integrity of my vaginal wall seemed worth it. But also, so much selling in pregnancy! Wasn't I meant to expand naturally? I never bought it.

I learned that certain postures could make tearing more likely. Namely, being supine with feet elevated in stirrups. I watched videos of people and animals giving birth. Elephants, gorillas, bears, giraffes. I saw a chimpanzee reach down and manually stretch her own perineum while laboring in a shoulder stand, hips skyward, legs dangling like pigtails. I watched many squatting births during which women looked centered, at ease. Our birth instructor explained that squatting cooperates with gravity. Perhaps we might choose this position if comfortable? I decided then and there that I would squat. It made sense.

I did not birth in a squatting pose. My labor was fast and hard, and then it was over. I didn't know that I had torn until I began to wonder what the midwife was doing down there, half an hour after my baby was born.

Stitching you up, she said.

I tore? I asked.

It's not bad, she said. Here's some ice.

I needed a wheelchair escort to recovery. Then help to the bathroom. Peeing burned. The on-call nurse brought me a numbing spray. I used it so liberally that she brought me another one later that day. I bled through pads and bed liners the size of picnic blankets, which I needed assistance to change. I didn't connect the stinging or bleeding to tearing. I thought this pain came with vaginal birth.

The odyssey continued after hospital discharge. I used a peri bottle to spray water on my vulva to dull the sting I felt when I peed. The pain was hot and sharp, momentarily soothed by sitting in a bowl of warm water that fit in the toilet seat, like a steamer basket hugging the pasta pot. A whiff of the lavender oil I sprinkled into the water can still remind me of doing that, the feeling of needles, the blood swirling through the water, my skin momentarily pinched by hard plastic. The bath provided relief, but preparing it felt so hard on top of round-the-clock breastfeeding and minimal sleep. I'm sure my mother or mother-in-law would have gladly helped me with this—they visited after the baby was born—but I was too ashamed to ask them. I could barely find the time to shower myself. Every walk around the block hurt. I thought what I was experiencing—the weeks of bleeding, the slow walking, the painful sitting—was how everyone healed from birth. That is, until I had my second baby. I walked perfectly, painlessly, from labor and delivery to recovery an hour afterward. Because that time, I didn't tear.

Months after my first birth, after the pain had stopped, I called the midwife to ask why I had torn. She barely remembered, but when she did, she said something about the baby zooming out, about my body failing to stretch. I was dissatisfied with what felt like a glib answer and angry that she didn't elaborate. Quickly the anger shapeshifted into self-blame. I blamed myself, or rather, I blamed my body, its lightening quick birth, for my tear. It was my fault; there was nothing to do.

Soon after that I began to wonder what the birth team hadn't done to prevent tearing. Or was something done that shouldn't have been? I called the midwifery practice again to ask for my records. The raspy voice on the other end told me I could fill out a consent form, and she would hand them over. The slim folder contained next to nothing. No record of repairing a tear. I still didn't know what part of my body tore. When I called back to ask why, the voice explained that the hospital keeps those records, not the midwife who caught my baby and sewed me back together.

I called the hospital records department. The man who answered told me to come in to sign a consent form. I walked over on a sweltering day that stank of trash. Filled out the form but didn't get the records, as I hadn't brought my driver's license, which I had recently misplaced. I would need to return with the license.

In the meantime, I noticed that my vulva looked different. Less like the smooth round place on a tree where a limb was removed, more asymmetric. It was as if my labia had separated and one had forked off. I asked another midwife who was caring for me at the time about it; she said she couldn't know exactly what had happened, but it looked like I had torn toward the front of my vulva, not back toward my posterior. After she confirmed that I wasn't experiencing any problems with sensation or function, she told me that this can happen, that the vulva's face can change after childbirth.

I couldn't share this with my mother, my aunt, and my grandmother in the kitchen. I hadn't processed it myself.

"SOME PEOPLE TEAR, AND SOME PEOPLE DON'T" IS A MYOPIC AND careless view of birthing bodies. Especially when we know providers can work to prevent tears.

The researchers at Evidence Based Birth gathered and synthesized the existing data on tear prevention and found five research-supported methods. The first is to avoid an episiotomy. The second, which I knew about from my childbirth class, is birth position. Supine positions, such as the traditional lithotomy position common at hospitals (half reclined, feet in stirrups), are associated with more perineal trauma and difficulty birthing than upright positions, such as sitting, squatting, and hands-and-knees. Perineal massage can help prevent tearing, especially when it's done gently and with a water-soluble lubricant during the second stage of labor. Putting pressure on the perineum with a warm, moist compress may also discourage tears. And lastly, tears can be avoided when doctors don't touch the perineum at all.

It's a relief to know that tearing prevention is possible. I wish I had known about these methods before giving birth. However, they are rarely used. Even worse, instead of helping their patients avoid tearing, doctors cause it.

Take positioning. Lying flat is the primary position birthers assume in US hospitals. More than 90 percent labor and birth on their backs or reclining in a hospital bed, the kind with foot stirrups. Only 4 percent squat or sit, 3 percent lie on their sides, and 1 percent are on hands and knees—all positions my birth class instructor recommended. As I learned about them, I wondered why positions that worked with gravity or seemed more comfortable for birthers themselves were so underused.

I remember entering a triage room and getting into the all-fours position on the gurney. But the staff didn't want me giving birth in there. They wanted me to go to a labor and delivery room. I couldn't walk there on my own—my labor was too intense. My baby was crowning. So they wheeled me into the room in the lithotomy position. By then I couldn't move, I couldn't choose. They encouraged me onto my back, my feet into the stirrups, and my daughter was born.

I had believed that in the hospital I would be able to choose the position I wanted to birth in, that I would have the capacity to telegraph my preference. Maybe no alternative birth position, no amount of midwifery skill, or even more knowledge on my part or different behavior could have altered my outcome. But position has been shown to protect against tearing. I wonder what would have happened if I had been allowed to birth in the shape my body wanted.

Many people labor and birth in a supine pose because it's easier for doctors, not for birthers. It allows doctors visibility, makes it easier for them to catch babies. This is why it persists. Doctors cajole or force women into their own preferred positions, even though they cause us to tear.

The next anti-tearing technique that Evidence Based Birth identi-fied is perineal massage with a lubricant during the second stage of labor. However, some hospital providers do it to women without ask-ing. They don't view perineal massage as something they need to get consent for. Consent isn't received "100 percent of the time in hospi-tals as far as I know," Dekker said. "That's terrible practice and could be traumatic. It's a medical procedure."

Labor and delivery unit workers shared that sometimes doctors use the mini bottles of baby shampoo that are lying around instead of a lubricant to perform the procedure. Inserting soap into the va-gina during labor is odious. "You're not supposed to put soap in there," Dekker said.

Another hands-on effort meant to reduce tearing is a warm moist towel held against the perineum during the second stage of labor. This technique reduces third- and fourth-degree tears by half, according to a literature review. It also decreases episiotomy use. But, oddly, re-searchers aren't exactly sure why the warm compress works to prevent tears—they don't know whether tears are reduced because the moist heat stretches the vaginal tissue, keeping the perineum intact, or be-cause applying the compress keeps doctors busy with a task so they don't cut you.

The final anti-tearing technique is to avoid touching the perineum at all or to touch it as minimally as possible. Some providers deliver aggressive hands-on care—meaning they're touching the perineum in some way, say, while doing an unskilled or aggressive perineal massage with baby soap—which leads to more severe tears and episiotomies.

The Instagram account Bad Ass Mother Birther, which has a his-tory of being censored on the platform for its childbirth content, once shared a post about what it called vaginal carving. "Let's talk about something that is often dismissed and has been integrated into birth as something that is passing as 'normal,'" the post begins. Provid-ers who insert their fingers into vaginas to "widen the space," "carve open the canal," "use fingers as forceps," and "rush the birth" are not practicing medicine. These actions are "often described by birthers as assault." Gwen Schroeder, a birth photographer and doula, has witnessed this.

"It looked like he was digging for gold," she said of one provider. She recalled the extreme discomfort of everyone in the room and lamented that nobody said anything. She thinks this was in part because he did it with the kind of authority that made it seem like an official procedure. Not only does this sweeping action constitute a violation of the birthing person, if done without consent, but it can also cause tearing.

The first and most important method to prevent tearing is avoiding an episiotomy in the first place. For generations, women—including my mother, aunt, and grandmother—never had a say in the matter. Episiotomy was a centerpiece of patriarchal medicine's twentieth-century push to control childbirth. Men drove its development and widespread use. Men whose perinea would remain inviolate, unthreatened by surgical scissors.

The technique for enlarging the baby's exit may have first been described in a 1742 midwifery text by a male midwife named Fielding Oud. "It is to be hoped that there is no Danger of hurting or destroying any Part, but just what necessity requires," Oud writes of what he calls "the incision," which he says should be "made as far as the prudent Operator thinks he may venture." Meaning that doctors should guess how much to cut.

This freewheeling kind of cutting hasn't benefited women. The perineal muscles spread so much that episiotomies often measure between two and four inches long. That's how much skin fans out. Doctors can cut so much that the rectal tissue or sphincter muscles can easily be torn or sliced. Overcutting is common. "This happens much more often than any doctor I've ever known cares to admit," writes Susan McCutcheon in *Natural Childbirth the Bradley Way*. After watching people give birth with more than one hundred different doctors, she said, "It has become apparent to me that the doctor's skill as a surgeon does not prevent [overcutting] from happening."

Cutting too much has awful ramifications. The pelvic floor muscle, the pubococcygeus, is the muscle you use to stop peeing; you also use it when climbing stairs, lifting anything with weight, and having vaginal intercourse. Using it feels like hugging yourself from the inside. Courtney Wyckoff, founder of the Momma Strong fitness community, whose exercises take a biomechanical approach to rehabilitation, describes moving the muscle as "blinking your pee hole and rocketing it up." Because the pubococcygeus surrounds the barrel of the vagina, it can very easily be incised unintentionally and then, because it is hidden, duck repair. Damage to this musculature is painful and threatens the organs, joints, and muscles involved in sitting, walking, and movement.

Episiotomy's pioneers believed that the surgery would save women's bodies from the supposed demolition that physiologic labor caused. Obstetrician Joseph DeLee had argued in the early 1900s that the procedure "restored virginal conditions" and that the mother, once stitched up, was then made "better than new." She and her body, flawed to start, were improved by him. DeLee promised that his medical arts birth protected babies too—and his methods likely wouldn't have gotten off of the ground without that addendum. DeLee warned that death by head trauma, brain damage, cerebral palsy, and even future criminal behavior were all risks of babies navigating the birth canal without help from surgeons. Episiotomy and forceps extraction rescued the baby from those horrible fates. For DeLee, a mother's body was a treacherous place. Comparing the damage childbirth did to women to falling on a pitchfork, he wondered why doctors would apply their techniques to one injury and not the other.

By prescribing a birth that required his presence and his tools, DeLee helped the obstetric profession paper over its failures, skirt censure, and prevent obsolescence. He enlivened the trade with a singular heroism, then persuaded women that they should search out that heroism in doctors since they lacked it themselves. Social historians Richard and Dorothy Wertz write that by the 1920s doctors believed that "normal" deliveries lacking the persistent "threat of tears in the women's perineum, were so rare as to be virtually nonexistent." And by the 1930s, DeLee's tear-proofing, sedation, and extraction birth had been mainstreamed into American hospitals. Birth became more "malleable, more a product of medical skill and technique," the

Wertzes write. DeLee's sedation necessitated episiotomy and forceps extraction because unconscious women couldn't push. As birth became a hospital procedure, episiotomy met it there.

DeLee wrought generational damage—"horrific impact on women's health for the next century," according to Dekker. Episiotomy record keeping was then and remains today very poor. We don't know much about its incidence until the late 1970s. This explains why generations of women—including in my own family—thought that being severed was required for their children to come out. Their doctors espoused cutting as necessary and routine, enlarging the space that, they believed, nature had failed to adequately size. They said straight lines heal better than jagged ones. That tearing was messy, while being sliced was clean. Nature was wrong and unkempt; technology was correct and pristine. This myth, articulated by male doctors, launched the procedure's use and abets its continued abuse. Episiotomy is hardly a relic of a bygone time. The World Health Organization estimates that it occurs in 60 percent of births today. Evidence Based Birth says rates are as high as 90 percent in parts of China, Thailand, and Latin America.

One would think that the near universal application of a surgery would require solid scientific support. With episiotomy, the opposite is true. A sweeping review of the literature on episiotomy comprising more than 350 books and articles published from 1860 to 1980 concluded that no science supports its widespread use. Zilch. Writing in 1983, when episiotomy was used in more than half of US births, researchers concluded, "There is no clearly defined evidence for its efficacy, particularly for routine use." They recommended clinical trials, as there had never been any.

The study that finally challenged episiotomy and led to its censure was a 1992 randomized controlled clinical trial that assigned 703 pregnant people either episiotomy or restricted use of the surgery. Doctors for the latter group struggled to avoid cutting people. They were so used to performing episiotomy that they couldn't stop, even when instructed to do so by researchers.

Still, the findings were stark. Forty-nine people who had episiotomies experienced severe tears, while only one person without an episiotomy did. Researchers discovered that episiotomy failed to prevent severe tearing, causing them to recommend that "liberal or routine use of episiotomy be abandoned." These were groundbreaking results, but researchers struggled to publish them in a respected journal because they contradicted what obstetricians were accustomed to doing in practice. Tradition was prized over evidence.

In 1995, the American College of Obstetricians and Gynecologists withdrew its support for the common cut. Additional research discovered that spontaneous tears hurt less than episiotomy-induced ones. The surgery not only fails to prevent perineal tears, incontinence, prolapse, and weakness, as DeLee promised, but causes these problems and others. A clinical trial in 2017 comparing selective episiotomy to its removal from birth entirely concluded that "the end of episiotomy is a goal that should be pursued within a humanized childbirth care model."

It's impossible to know how often episiotomies are cut today. Hospital rates swing between 1 and 40 percent, according to the Leapfrog Group, a nonprofit healthcare watchdog. The massive range "suggests that some doctors still perform the snip even when it may not be necessary," explained a 2019 report in the *New York Times*. "Snip" is infantilization, as we haven't reckoned with what the surgery is and the damage it does. Tellingly, another study found that the longer an obstetrician practices, the higher his episiotomy rate, suggesting that, as with other procedures, tradition, not evidence, propels episiotomy use.

Hospitals know their own rates—episiotomies are surgical procedures they are required to catalogue—but most refuse to share them publicly. Episiotomies are included in data used to set insurance premiums, and they factor into hospital performance grades. Hospitals are disincentivized from reporting high numbers. Birthers—who, let's remember, are consumers—enter the hospital blind to all of this.

"In every other hospital unit, we have crazy measures in place to prevent breaking skin—as we should," Barbie Christianson, a labor and delivery nurse, told me. She went on to stress that in the birth ward skin gets broken more aggressively, and unnecessarily often.

Many birth professionals who believe the procedure amounts to genital mutilation stop short of calling it that. It should never happen without consent, but it often does. More than one-fifth of moms responding to the 2013 Listening to Mothers survey had an episiotomy, yet 59 percent of them said they did not consent to being cut. Some mentioned that healing from their episiotomy was a grisly process. More than 60 percent of those who shared about their episiotomy in my survey had not been aware that their doctor was performing one or did not consent to the procedure, which tracks with the Listening to Mothers data.

"I don't remember it being a question," said Paige of her episiotomy in Brooklyn in 2014. "I don't remember if she told me she was doing it or if she just did it. I didn't opt in." "I was given an episiotomy and didn't even know it! My OB just did it," Heather in Arlington, Illinois, said. Annsley in New York had told her obstetrician in prenatal appointments that she really didn't want one, but he did one anyway. "He didn't even discuss with me afterward why he opted to give me one," she explained. Andrea in Greensboro, North Carolina, wasn't asked beforehand or even told afterward. "I felt him stitching me up and he said, 'You can feel that,' and numbed it some more," she said. "That's how I found out he made the incision, and I had specifically told them I did not want one."

"If a doctor does act upon them without their consent, that's a battery," Hermine Hayes-Klein told me. She is one of the few lawyers in the US who represent victims in obstetric violence cases. But it's not being called battery, abuse, or assault in the cultural conversation. Reports often frame an episiotomy done without consent as a missed opportunity for women to make a choice, not as illegal abuse suffered during childbirth.

Episiotomies persist because doctors swear they're necessary, that the incision is prevention. They say, this is an emergency, we have to cut to save you, to save your baby. They might tell you this is "what a good mom does" or frighten you: "You don't want to harm your baby." Often they have already administered drugs that numb from the waist down, so you can't listen to your body to know what to do. Birthing people fear tearing, so we acquiesce. As Susan McCutcheon put it, "Doctors say this is the way they were taught and this is the way they do it; it works for them and they don't know any other way—and, frankly, it doesn't hurt them a bit."

Not surprisingly, two of the greatest predictors of tearing are provider and birth setting. A study comparing obstetric and midwifery care found that homes and birth centers have lower rates of the most common tears than hospitals. You're more likely to tear giving birth in the hospital than in a birth center or at home. Geography may matter too. Midwifery programs in the United Kingdom and Europe boast extremely low or nonexistent perineal laceration rates. Across the pond, they support and protect perinea.

Midwives are more likely to do things to prevent tears than doctors, and they're also less likely to use episiotomy, forceps, and vacuums, all implements associated with tears. All of my survey respondents' episiotomies were performed by obstetricians. Dekker found in the research that while all the evidence-based methods for tear prevention were good, studies of experienced midwives seemed to prove that what they know and do in the birth room prevents tearing better than any of the individual actions providers take alone.

A study of twelve experienced certified nurse midwives in New Mexico found that in 1,211 births, 73 percent required no stitching, and the severe tear rate was between .7 and 1.5 percent. Only ten episiotomies were cut. These results were impressive, far better than what's standard, leading many to wonder how they did it. The findings dovetailed with what expert midwives in Ireland and New Zealand shared when asked about how they maintained such low tear and suture rates.

Midwives' cumulative years of experience and knowledge provide the answer. Their success in preventing tears was less about exercising a menu of actions than the culture they created around the birth. It was calm and slow. The midwives supported the birthers in non-Valsalva, spontaneous pushing—meaning they didn't hold their breath, and they pushed with their own urges rather than on a doctor's command. Position matters—80 percent of those giving birth did so sitting upright. The head and shoulders were birthed slowly and gently. The midwives encouraged women to laugh, cough, giggle, blow, participate in the labor sensations, and match them with any actions that might help. The midwives noticed the color of the perineal tissue. If it was losing blood and turning white, meaning it could tear, they slowed down and only suggested pushing when the skin had returned to pink. They shepherded birthers through the body's natural process.

Who touches birthing people matters. A retrospective study of more than fifteen thousand births discovered that experienced midwives had lower rates of severe tears using hands-on care, and the decreased risk to birthing people shot up with each additional year of practical experience the midwife had. The takeaway is that experienced, skillful midwives using hands can prevent tears, while doctors cause them. Hospitals deploy aggressive perineal massage and episiotomy. Midwives' skilled and holistic experience using massage prevents tears and aids birth.

By the time I obtain my medical records, the baby whose birth precipitated my tear is nearly seven years old. The hospital halls are dim and smell like sanitizer and cafeteria food. The chipper employee behind the Plexiglas tells me they'll be emailed at a small cost, payable to a third party online.

Anything that happened while you were here will be in there, she assures me. Within ten business days.

I sanitize my hands at one of the many freestanding pumps in a large hall. I catch sight of a flyer offering breastfeeding advice in ten steps. Then I pass a wall of 1920s portraits featuring groups of nurses posed like sorority sisters. They all wear white dresses, pointy hats, solemn stares. I wonder how many episiotomies they saw.

Because the tissues are engorged with blood from birth when they are repaired, vulvas can heal asymmetrically and appear different from before. Kimberly Johnson, a body worker and author of a book about the fourth trimester, who tore during childbirth, advises her patients to take photos of their vulvas before they have babies, so they can remember what they look like. One woman brought it to her birth "so if she needed a repair, her midwife or doctor would know how she looked originally and help to return her as close as possible to how she was," Johnson explains. I wonder if they could have waited until the swelling went down to sew me up. Had I brought a picture, would it have changed anything?

The email with my report goes into my junk folder. I dig it out and download the file of my two childbirths at the hospital, which clocks in at 188 pages. I begin to read, then realize how much of it doesn't relate to what I hope to learn, how much of it is internal jargon or pro forma advice about healing from vaginal birth and identifying postpartum depression. I find "Other specified trauma to perineum and vulva during delivery," then I keyword search "tear," "laceration," and "repair."

On page thirty-five I find the most information about this that I'm going to get. "Vaginal Lacerations: Periurethral Laceration, Repaired. Labial Laceration, Repaired." Some follow-up internet research tells me that both of these kinds of tears, tears of the vulva, are often not stitched up and frequently do heal on their own. One expert recommends keeping legs closed for a couple of weeks to coax the tissues back together. I vaguely remember asking what degree tear I had, as I lay there and felt the tugging beneath, my baby's crinkly skin sticking to my chest. The midwife was focused on the stitches.

It's not that bad, she had said.

I also affirm what I experienced—pain, discomfort, a change in the way I look. What does it mean to know this now? Nothing has changed beyond the appearance of my anatomy.

I had first-degree tears in two places. First-degree tears supposedly do not need repair and are not so painful, but that was not my experience. Healing from them was very painful, at times miserable. Enough so that I was angry and wondered what could have been done to prevent them. I continue to wonder. Maybe many things. Maybe nothing. But I am grateful to know now what generations of women before me didn't. That cutting doesn't save you from pain. That cutting without consent can be considered assault. Sharing this now gives me hope that the touch we receive in birth can be what we deserve: gentle, skilled, and welcome.

CHAPTER 6
SURGICAL STRIKE

PICTURE THE MAGIC TRICK THAT FEATURES A MAN, A WOMAN, A long box, and blades. She's inside, but the audience can only see the crown of her head, hair cascading down. The magician inserts the blades through the box at her chest and stomach. Then he pushes the boxes apart.

This is how LaToya Jordan describes the birth of her daughter in the spring of 2012. Lying in the box, chopped into thirds, her midsection extracted from the rest of her. The genders of the trick's participants seem predetermined—male magician, female subject—and mirror the power dynamics in the surgery responsible for one-third of births in the United States.

Put simply, a cesarean is an operation lasting about forty-five minutes. A spinal block injection numbs below the neck. Then the surgeon cuts an incision above the pubic hair line, opening the skin, muscles, and fat of the abdomen, along with the corn-husk-like layers of fascia that buoy the stomach's contents. Then the uterus is exposed, and the baby is removed. Neel Shah, an OBGYN at Harvard who has performed thousands of C-sections, said that at this point, "The baby very quickly becomes the most interesting thing in the room. Then you very carefully put everything back the way you found it."

C-sections have a colorful and gruesome backstory spanning thousands of years. The cesarean's nomenclature honors the men who ordained its use, rather than the women who endured it. The practice goes back to ancient Rome, where, according to tradition, the city's second king, Numa Pompilius, ordered that fetuses be removed from uteruses when mothers were dying or dead. This pronouncement, issued possibly as early as the eighth century BCE, became *Lex caesarea*, or royal law. There is no evidence for the common story that Julius Caesar was born this way.

Historically, the procedure was used to preserve royal bloodlines. As recently as the twentieth century, Germans called the surgery *Kaiserschnitt* after their emperors, Kaisers. When a mother was gravely ill or had died, a baby was cut out in an attempt to save him (not her) and the patriarchal lineage. Later incarnations of the procedure continued to sacrifice mothers to save the unborn. Religious scholars in the 1700s favored babies over mothers because babies needed baptism to save their souls from purgatory, whereas adult women were heaven ready. In 1930, Pope Pius XI forbade doctors from ending a baby's life to save its mother, spiking C-section rates and maternal mortality at a time when the surgery was still quite dangerous.

In the US, the first successful C-section—as in, the first C-section in which the mother survived—likely occurred in 1794, in a rural, unsterile cabin in what is now West Virginia. Jesse Bennett believed his laboring wife, Elizabeth, might die, so he sidestepped the family doctor and operated on her himself after dosing her with the opium tincture laudanum, which put her to sleep. He also removed her ovaries, according to one account, saying later he "would not be subjected to such an ordeal again." Elizabeth and her child survived, but the historical record doesn't include how she felt about waking up without ovaries, having gone to sleep without agreeing to their removal. Later, in 1876, an Italian professor recommended that cesareans routinely include hysterectomies, to prevent the hemorrhaging that many women experienced before suture use was widespread.

The cesarean was invented to save babies' lives, but it does so today only in incredibly rare circumstances. The vast majority of C-sections are performed for other reasons, and the surgery is overused to a shocking degree. Cesarean birth is blindly assumed for many pregnancy conditions, when it might not be required at all. Furthermore, pregnant people might actively reject surgery but aren't able to exercise informed consent and refusal. They have no choice and are often coerced. Hospitals and individual doctors who overuse this surgery aren't doing so out of an abundance of caution or medical necessity. They are practicing (and sustaining and rationalizing) an ancient form of social control.

In the 1970s, the C-section rate in the US was around 5 percent. Today it's almost 32 percent—a 500 percent increase. The World Health Organization recommends a C-section rate of between 10 and 15 percent for a healthy population; America's is more than twice that. Other countries' rates are worse. Mexico's is 50 percent for first-time mothers. Brazil's private hospitals C-section up to 90 percent of the time.

Why the high rates? The blame often falls on birthing people themselves. Rather than wait to go into labor, women schedule babies to arrive at their convenience. Famous white women allegedly sought "designer" C-sections because they were controlling (Madonna) or lazy (Kate Hudson). Victoria Beckham was reportedly "too Posh to push," scheduling her three C-sections around her husband's soccer calendar. Elective C-sections are "clear evidence of the self-obsessed behavior exhibited by some celebrity mothers finding new ways to push the narcissistic envelope," according to one (white, male) commentator. Condemning women may be appealing, but elective C-sections are a very small fraction of the total—around 2 percent; they're definitely not driving the increase.

People wonder if it even matters that C-sections are overused. After all, the procedure has been perfected in recent decades. It's the most common surgery in the US, with more than a million of them per-formed every year. The fact that they're routine must mean they are needed and safe. In the majority of US hospitals, cesareans are com-pulsory for breech babies and multiples, and encouraged for pregnant women over age thirty-five, diabetics, and those who have been told they're carrying big babies.

As Wayne Cohen, a former hospital chief of obstetrics, asked me, "If we can maximize good outcomes, does it matter whether we ac-complish that goal with a cesarean rate of 10 percent or 30 percent?" I guess it depends on your definition of a good outcome and whether you value the well-being and will of women. Or, as the obstetrician Neel Shah put it, "Women have goals in labor other than emerging unscathed. Survival and not being cut open is the floor. We should be designing a system that's aimed at the ceiling."

IF YOU WERE TO PLOT THE C-SECTION RATES OF AMERICAN HOSPI-tals on a graph and connect the dots, you would basically have a Jack-son Pollack or something drawn by my three-year-old. They are all over the place, ranging from 7 to 70 percent. The best predictors of whether or not a pregnant person will undergo a C-section are the hospital's rate, the doctor's rate, and race. Essentially, zip codes, not underlying conditions, determine the spread.

Hospitals and doctors with high C-section rates like the conve-nience of it. Surgical delivery is far more predictable and manageable than vaginal delivery. Vaginal delivery requires birth attendants to essentially wait and do nothing. Waiting and doing nothing are not in obstetricians' training. They're masters of acting. A large study of more than twenty-one thousand birth records from seventy-two hospitals in sixteen states identified an uptick in first-time C-sections during three times of day: morning, lunch, and early evening. An-other study found the majority of operations occur between 9 a.m. and 5 p.m. Doctors perform sections when it's convenient for them. They don't want to work late.

You can't talk about a medical procedure in America without mentioning its cost. For a routine yet complicated surgery like a C-section, the cost is high, and the incentives for performing as many of them as possible are therefore great. The numbers are hard to come by, but some figures have become public after being hidden for years. A 2021 *Wall Street Journal* investigation found that at the Van Ness campus of Sutter Health's California Pacific Medical Center, a C-section could cost as much as $60,584. Other hospitals charged as little as $6,241, or $29,257, or $38,264. Medicaid patients usually paid under $10,000, while out-of-network private plans paid more than $40,000. A friend in Seattle had a $30,000 C-section, thankfully covered by her insurance. C-sections are costly in other countries too. In Mexico's private hospitals, they can cost five times as much as vaginal deliveries.

"We make crazy money off of C-section, infection, and complicated birth. Every hospital does," Kavita Patel, a former executive at Johns Hopkins Medicine's Sibley Memorial Hospital, one of the country's largest hospital systems, told me. "We made such little money in Medicaid that we barely wanted to take it."

Pricey C-sections have driven up the cost of all hospital births. As part of the leadership team for eight years, Patel negotiated with insurance companies to secure the best coverage rates for services at her hospital. Vaginal births are costly too, not because they require expensive medical intervention but because of how they are classified for insurance purposes.

"Even the vaginal delivery is billed as a surgery," Patel told me. "Because you're using a surgical suite. If you ever wondered why, when labor and delivery wings are full, why we can't put those pregnant women into regular hospital rooms? It's because all these labor and delivery rooms are outfitted to convert into operating rooms if we need them to." That is, if patients suddenly needed C-sections. "That comes with a prenegotiated facility fee," Patel continues. "Blue Cross Blue Shield agrees to pay me more for that room than a person with pneumonia in another room."

The moneymaking is not only in the facilities but also in the churn. "Little pregnant women on an assembly line" was how one colleague put it to Patel. "That's really what it is. The more people we can get in and out of the door, the more money I can make." And there's no incentive to change that. Improvements that aren't drugs and tools—providing support and comfort measures, allowing a birthing person to move around and eat and drink, and supporting physiologic birth—are often denied or rejected on the basis of policy and procedure or because of a false claim that they're dangerous. In reality, it's because they give more time and control to patients, and that reduces a hospital's bottom line.

Patel put it bluntly: "Even though patients and pregnant people would benefit, improvements for women lose money.... Maternity is the best moneymaker. It really is."

Race, alongside money, is another reliable predictor of medical procedures and outcomes. The C-section rate has recently dipped slightly for white women, but it has increased for Black women. A 2021 Centers for Disease Control and Prevention report found a 35.9 percent C-section rate for Black women, the highest for any group in the US. Meanwhile, Black women and infants continue to experience the highest incidence of poor birth outcomes—prematurity and mortality among them. The link between this tragedy and C-sections is infrequently discussed.

C-SECTION MISINFORMATION ABOUNDS. SOME OF IT IS ROOTED IN myth, believed and perpetuated by doctors and hospitals, some of it results from bad or outdated research, and some of it is social construction. But whatever the reason for them, the falsehoods produce terrible consequences for women.

Sylvia Guendelman, a professor of public health at the University of California, Berkeley, found that pregnant people often believe more technology is better and safer when it comes to childbirth. The thinking is "if you're in the hands of a doctor who does C-sections, you're going to be in better hands," Guendelman told me. When I asked

Shah about this, he said the whole concept of more technology being better for childbirth is absolutely untrue. That's because "compared to normal delivery, the odds of suffering a major complication of birth, like hemorrhage, sepsis, organ injury, things that are life-threatening, are about three times more likely to occur with a C-section than without one," he said.

The other reason C-sections aren't inherently safer is because of the increasing difficulty of the surgery when a pregnant person has already had one before. Cesareans create scar tissue inside the abdomen, which can lead to the placenta burrowing into the uterine wall, a condition called accreta. Placenta accreta rates have climbed alongside C-sections, quadrupling since the 1980s. You may have heard that Kim Kardashian had it. The diagnosis, formerly part of a group of placental conditions called morbidly adherent placenta, presents a severe bleeding risk during and after birth. It can be life-threatening or cause infertility. The American College of Obstetricians and Gynecologists (ACOG) and the Society for Maternal-Fetal Medicine recommend that doctors have quick access to blood-transfusion resources for accreta patients. The most common risk factor for accreta is a previous C-section.

Another pervasive myth is that C-section preserves sexual attractiveness and pleasure, whereas vaginal birth threatens them. Rio de Janeiro boasts one of the highest C-section rates on earth; there, "90 percent of wealthy women would rather pay for the operation than put their vaginas at risk," according to Tina Cassidy, who herself had a C-section and researched them for *Birth: The Surprising History of How We Are Born*.

But birth does not threaten vaginal integrity or pleasurable sex. "There is a prevailing notion among some cultures and some people that normal vaginal delivery can disrupt sexual function. There's absolutely no scientific evidence that that's the case," Shah said. "It sounds awfully socially constructed as an idea, right?"

Guendelman found in her research that women in Mexico City were drawn to C-section because they think "sex is better, pain lower, it's quicker, and I can have it whenever I want." This idea dovetails with another misconception: that C-sections are less painful than vaginal births. Although the harder recovery associated with C-section—one must recover from both birth and surgery—would seem to disprove this, Guendelman hears this claim repeatedly from her study subjects. Even some doctors believe this, so the myth goes unchallenged.

Planning something can seem easier than waiting for the unknown, and convenience is often a reason cited for scheduling a C-section. But Shah and other advocates of reducing C-sections believe that perceived short-term convenience isn't worth the long-term risk. Guendelman saw that in Mexico "providers lack patience with the labor process," a finding that leads to more C-sections. Meanwhile, she believes that Mexican birthers should develop a stronger consumer voice in the delivery room, similar to the one she has seen emerging in the US in the past decade. She hopes to see more Mexican women questioning the C-section norm.

"It's another way of performing violence against women," she said.

ANOTHER PERVASIVE C-SECTION MYTH IS THAT THEY ARE RE-quired to deliver breech babies. Breech means a baby's head is presenting in a direction other than downward, toward the vaginal opening, near the end of a pregnancy. The baby may be presenting feet or buttocks first, for example.

Breech babies shouldn't be automatic C-sections. Safe breech vaginal birth is as old as birth itself, and it used to be the norm as recently as the 1970s, when the C-section rate was much lower than it is today. Breech births are often compulsory C-sections now because very few obstetricians today can deliver breech babies vaginally. They are trained to perform cesareans, not to support vaginal delivery, to wait for and catch a baby arriving feet first.

The dissolution of this obstetric capability can essentially be traced to a single study, published more than twenty years ago. In the Term Breech Trial, led by Mary E. Hannah at the University of Toronto, 2,088 pregnant women carrying breech babies were randomly assigned to deliver vaginally or through C-section. These women gave birth in 121 facilities across twenty-six countries. Researchers found no difference in maternal outcomes for either group but reported that the risk to babies was "significantly lower" if they were delivered surgically. The authors used this finding to advise that "planned caesarean section is better than planned vaginal birth for the term fetus in the breech presentation." As another researcher, Molly Dickens, put it to me, "They basically state, 'It just isn't worth it, do the C-section.'"

Because its results were published in the prestigious medical journal *The Lancet* in 2000, the reach of the study cannot be overstated. Entire countries changed how they managed birth. Although Dickens wasn't involved in the study, she analyzed it closely. She said that the Netherlands increased its C-section rate for breech babies from 50 to 80 percent within two months of the study's publication. Others have criticized the study, and *The Lancet* published a follow up. "An option of no option, in which breech presentation ... automatically indicates caesarean section with no alternative, seems too alluring to resist. The unintended consequence has been an increase in maternal morbidity and mortality, especially in low-resource settings," wrote Jos van Roosmalen, a professor of global health, and Tarek Meguid, an OBGYN, in *The Lancet* in 2014. The "condemnation of vaginal breech delivery by one randomized controlled trial" has had a "sweeping effect on clinical practice," according to another critique, by Andrew Kotsaka, that was published in the *British Medical Journal*. Tellingly, the US C-section rate has ballooned ever since the original Term Breech Trial findings were made public. The trial continues to influence the deliveries and lives of moms.

Eradicating vaginal delivery for breech babies based on a single study is ethically dubious. While randomized clinical trials are thought to produce the strongest scientific evidence, they can also have serious limitations. Applying their results to individuals is tricky. In the Term Breech Trial, Kotsaka pointed out, low-risk breech pregnancies were lumped together with higher-risk ones. The ability of experienced obstetricians to make judgment calls about whether to deliver vaginally or by C-section was not taken into account. The trial forced practitioners to "exceed their comfort level," delivering some breech babies vaginally who, in their clinical opinion, might have needed C-sections, and others via C-section who might have been safer with a vaginal delivery. They were more or less forced to perform emergency cesareans when, in a typical hospital setting, they might have deemed it unnecessary. Because of the study, obstetricians began automatically performing C-sections in breech presentations instead of developing and applying their skills and judgment to the specific details of each case.

Critics from Australia, Belgium, Canada, France, Israel, the Netherlands, and Norway have raised alarms about the eradication of vaginal breech delivery, due to the Term Breech Trial. Such critiques have appeared in prestigious medical journals and have been aired for years. Critics take issue with the study for not following the postoperative and long-term consequences for C-sections—only measuring outcomes in the immediate weeks after the births, rather than farther into the future, before publishing their findings. The researchers did, however, continue to follow a subgroup of children born in the trial, and in 2003, led this time by Hilary Whyte, they published their findings: death and abnormal neurodevelopment were similar among children in the two groups. In other words, those born via C-section *weren't* found to be better off than those born vaginally, as the trial authors had originally stated.

Whether a pregnant person desires (or refuses or fears) surgical or vaginal birth should lead discussions about how to approach birth, but this is uncommon. "You wouldn't be comfortable having a general surgeon remove a brain tumor, right?" Dickens asks. It's similar with breech birth. Birthing people might opt for cesarean birth instead of vaginal birth if there isn't someone with the knowledge to do the latter safely. But in nearly all cases, women aren't given a choice. By varying degrees, they're forced or coerced into a surgery they may not want or need.

A handful of doctors who can deliver breech babies vaginally do exist, but they don't tend to advertise that they will do the procedure. Referrals are more word-of-mouth. A friend of mine in North Carolina looked for one and said she could find only a single doctor in her entire state willing to *possibly* attend a breech vaginal labor, depending on which type of breech position her baby was in on her delivery date.

When doing handstands in a swimming pool didn't turn her daughter, Gwen, another friend of mine, called obstetricians across New York to find someone qualified and willing to attend a vaginal breech birth. "The only two that would do it were in their sixties, the old school method of delivery, and they didn't accept insurance," she told me. "We had to make this choice. Are we going to be out of pocket $20,000 in order to have this experience that we had wanted for ourselves?" Even if you can locate someone who is qualified, with that high a cost, vaginal breech delivery isn't a choice most people can make.

WOMEN CARRYING MULTIPLE BABIES ARE ALMOST ALWAYS GIVEN C-sections. Rates of cesarean twin births in the US rose from 55 percent in 1995 to over 75 percent in 2008. In Germany in 2012, 77 percent of twin births were surgical. But it doesn't have to be this way.

When Erica Rice found out she was pregnant with twins, she began discussing a vaginal birth with her OBGYN. She wanted a twin vaginal birth after cesarean. VBACs in general are withheld or frowned upon in American hospitals today, but twin VBACs are almost unheard of. Both twins were in the head-down position at thirty-eight weeks when Erica's water broke, and through what she called "a Herculean team effort," her twins were born vaginally at Boston's Beth Israel Deaconess Medical Center in 2017. She maintains that the birth wouldn't have been possible without her strong desire to have it and her providers' support and knowledge.

A vaginal birth of her twins wasn't even on Kelsey Mooseker's radar. "I just assumed I would have a scheduled C-section. That's what you do," she told me. But her provider, Bettina Paek, surprised her when she checked the babies' positions toward the end of Kelsey's pregnancy and asked, "What do you think about a vaginal birth if they are head down?"

"To put it on the table was amazing," Kelsey told me. This was the first time I had heard of a provider recommending a vaginal birth to a twin mom. With Paek's support, Kelsey birthed her twins vaginally in 2019 at Evergreen Health Family Maternity Center in Kirkland, Washington.

Both twin births were second pregnancies, and both women delivered in hospitals that were committed to and working toward lowering their C-section rates. The women benefited from the guidance and support of skilled doctors who informed them and treated them as experts in their own labor and birth.

In recent years, for the first time ever, women in their thirties, like Kelsey, are having more babies than women in their twenties. But birthing older doesn't oblige intervention, despite the widely held cultural belief that it does. Age itself isn't a risk factor. And yet, pregnancies in people thirty-five and older are stigmatized and shepherded toward risky intervention, beginning with the very terminology used to describe them. Designations like "geriatric pregnancy," "advanced maternal age," and even "elderly pregnancy" belong in the garbage bin. These connotations likely contribute to more cesareans in older demographics: 37 percent of pregnant people thirty-five to thirty-nine have C-sections, while 70 percent of those forty-five to forty-nine do, per ACOG. But those thirty-five and older who schedule C-sections face double the risk of severe maternal morbidity, according to a study in a Canadian medical journal. OBGYN Robyn Horsager-Boehrer believes women over thirty-five are electing to have C-sections without understanding their inherent risks—hemorrhage, stroke, blood clots, major organ dysfunction, and intensive care unit admission. "It's important for women thirty-five and older to carefully consider whether the convenience of a scheduled delivery is worth risking their health or even their lives," she wrote. It is the *procedure* that is laden with serious risk, not the bodies of those who have it.

C-section is perhaps most commonly assumed necessary if a woman has already had one. Once a C-section, always a C-section, the thinking goes. But that thinking, too, is flawed. Neel Shah says that even if you've had two previous C-sections, "you can still labor normally and that might be the best thing for you." ACOG recommends a VBAC because it dodges the risks of surgery and because most pregnant people are good candidates. But its guidelines are being ignored. Too often, providers couch VBAC in scary language or otherwise discourage it. Often pregnant people don't even know it's possible because their providers don't mention it at all.

C-SECTIONS ARE ABSOLUTELY NEEDED, ACCORDING TO SHAH, IN A few rare scenarios that endanger mom and baby: placenta previa, when the placenta covers the cervix; vasa previa, when fetal blood vessels move into the uterus, putting it at risk of rupture; and umbilical cord prolapse, when the umbilical cord drops into the vagina and blocks the baby's exit. These needed C-sections make up only about 4 percent of the total. The other 96 percent are, by Shah's definition, unnecessary.

Any surgery, even if common or relatively safe, bears inherent risk. But it's inappropriate to compare risks associated with C-section to the risks posed by other surgeries, as is often done, since you can't choose another kind of surgery to birth a baby. C-section is it. C-section risks should be compared to vaginal birth risks. And the odds of suffering a serious or life-threatening complication are three times greater with a C-section than with physiologic birth.

The recovery from a C-section is more difficult than that from a vaginal birth. Vaginal births heal relatively quickly by comparison. "I've examined a lot of people after they've given birth normally, just a couple of weeks later in the office," Shah told me. "That part of the body is actually designed to heal very quickly. In many cases there would be no way of knowing that somebody had a baby just a few weeks earlier."

After a C-section, in contrast, most women report that they can't lift their babies immediately after the procedure and are warned against picking up anything heavier than a car seat for six weeks. (And someone else should ideally lift that car seat.) The surgery makes basic movement harder, not to mention the new responsibilities of caring for an infant. It can disrupt milk production and make latching and breastfeeding more challenging. If there is no nursery in the hospital and a woman doesn't have a partner, or if the partner is not present, the new mother can hardly care for herself, let alone the baby. Scar pain after the operation, pelvic floor weakness or discomfort, and incontinence can occur.

Shah points out that a cesarean is the only procedure in which surgeons reopen the same scar. Most first C-sections are relatively straightforward, while subsequent ones are riskier. "I've done surgeries where it feels like I'm operating on a melted box of crayons," Shah said. Many people have more than one kid. And the risks increase with each C-section. Some providers recommend that their C-section birthers limit their family size.

The strongest case for lowering the C-section rate is its unspoken role in the maternal mortality crisis. "An American mom today is 50 percent more likely to die in childbirth than her own mom was. We're doing generational damage," Shah said. Black women are three to four times more likely to die than white women. Many deaths are preventable. C-section is central to this tragedy but omitted from the conversation, despite the risks of maternal death and severe complications that it carries in comparison to vaginal birth.

Three leading causes of maternal mortality are postpartum hemorrhage (11 percent), sepsis (13 percent), and hypertensive disorders such as preeclampsia (11 percent), according to the global nonprofit Patient Safety Movement Foundation. Together, these conditions account for about 35 percent of deaths in postpartum moms. Cesareans can cause or increase the risk of them all.

None of this is discussed when a C-section is ordered. That term—ordered—is fitting. The procedure is almost always framed as either an emergency or an absolute necessity. "The question of who actually needs a C-section is really hard," Shah told me. "Because in hindsight everyone who got one seems like they needed it. What I mean by that is personally when I do a C-section, it seems like I'm always right because if the baby comes out and looks perfect, you think, 'Well, it's a good thing I did a C-section. The baby looks perfect.' And if the baby comes out and looks kind of blue and lackluster, you think, 'That was a sick baby. It's a good thing I did a C-section.' Either way it's pretty good to be me because I'm always right."

C-section risk is a term levied like a parking ticket, from exam rooms to current research studies. We're told that many factors are correlated with C-section risk, like fetal head size, maternal age, prior C-section history, fetal distress, whether you're carrying multiples, and if you've had a surgical birth before. "They'll say, 'The risk of C-section' as if it's, like, naturally happening to a woman," Holly Dunsworth, the anthropologist, told me. "Instead of saying 'the risk that a medical professional will decide to intervene.'" It's not the same as one's risk of getting sick—of catching Covid, or the flu. "This is a human deciding I want to cut this baby out of this lady because I'm tired of waiting or I'm worried for her. And yet it's framed like it's just inevitable for her. It's a human decision."

LIKE WOMEN FOR MILLENNIA, LATOYA JORDAN'S RELATIONSHIP to childbirth had been a mashup of fascination and horror. "I thought it would be the hardest thing that I did but also the greatest experience. Like a life-changing moment that I would remember until the day I die," she told me. I wanted to talk to LaToya about her C-section after she described it in an anthology titled *My Caesarean*. "As a writer, I try to spin my trauma into beautiful scenes," she explains. "Symbols help me cope. It's the way I sort out my feelings."

When she was pregnant, LaToya watched every YouTube video of childbirth she could find. Her favorite was in water. "I wanted to look like these women," she told me. "At the end they just scooped their babies up out of the water, and it looked so beautiful." Every time she watched the literal moment a woman became a mother—the guttural yell, the body flail, and then her hungry arms clutching a gooey newborn to her breast, LaToya cried and longed for her turn. She read books, polled her friends, studied hypnobirthing, hired a doula, and attended prenatal yoga classes. The possibility of cesarean didn't enter her mind. LaToya knew what she wanted and how to refuse what she didn't, and her husband and doula were at her side.

LaToya awoke when her water broke—"like a balloon bursting." She and her husband jumped out of bed and grabbed the box of

Depends. She put one on for the thirty-minute trip from her home in Bedford-Stuyvesant to the birthing center. Her doula met them there. LaToya was examined in the waiting room because the birthing suites were occupied. The midwife recommended she transfer to the hospital when she found meconium "the color of split pea soup" in LaToya's amniotic fluid, suggesting an infection. LaToya had already been in labor for about nine hours when she transferred to a New York City hospital where more than eight thousand babies are born each year. She later learned that it had the highest birthrate in the entire city. When she arrived, every seat in the waiting room was taken. LaToya labored on the sidewalk for an hour. She had imagined an outdoor birth that was more woodland fairy, less garbage bins and taxis. But here she was, doubled over a bench, breathing in the stench of city asphalt. "Not what I pictured," she said.

LaToya was finally ushered into an exam room that was so small her doula and husband had to remain standing. "They attached me to the fetal heart rate monitor, and I was in the room for hours. They would come in to check on me but not a lot. Maybe every hour?" LaToya felt her baby pressing on her bladder. "It felt like every fifteen minutes she would unhook me from the machine, take me to the bathroom, bring me back, and hook me back up. We did that over and over and over again for hours."

LaToya declined the Pitocin offered to speed up her contractions. "If I have Pitocin, that's the beginning of the end of what I want to happen," she told me. LaToya had read about the "cascade of interventions" that can occur and often culminate in an unnecessary C-section. Finally, after some cajoling, which included being warned that she wasn't very dilated but her baby's heart rate was elevating, LaToya agreed to Pitocin. The contractions quickly became unbearable. "I'm on the conveyor belt, and I'm moving toward this birth that I read about," she recalled thinking.

LaToya remembers finding out that the obstetrician was planning to give her a C-section when the woman's hand was in her vagina. The doctor was examining her and asked, "How did you get that scar? Is it hypertonic or keloid?" LaToya has a scar on her face, slight as a pencil mark, from a car accident when she was a teen. The doctor told her, "Well, you're going to have a C-section, and I'm just wondering how the scar is going to heal."

"That was the first mention of C-section," LaToya said. "Her fingers are in my vagina. She's asking me these questions. I'm like, 'This is weird.'" LaToya remembers the doctor shaking her head "as if I were a child and had a skinned knee," she later wrote. Another obstetrician had mistaken her husband for her boyfriend, even though she had introduced him as her spouse, making her wonder whether the doctor confused white women's partners in the same way.

Moya Bailey, a communications professor at Northwestern University, who studies the intersection of race, gender, and sexuality, created the term *misogynoir* to refer to the specific, race-based misogyny that is directed toward Black women in popular culture, but it's a useful term in the context of birth too. "Sometimes you can't tear them apart—like sexism and racism are joined together in my experience," LaToya said.

Two hospital practices cause the most unnecessary C-sections—one is a diagnosis; the other, a tool. They are worth unpacking because they are complicated and because misogyny and misogynoir reside at their root. The first is "failure to progress," which is diagnosed when labor appears to stall. *Arrest of labor* and *dystocia* are the clinical terms, but the outdated, judgmental-sounding "failure to progress" is still ubiquitous.

The "failure to progress" diagnosis can be traced to Columbia University obstetrician Emanuel Friedman's 1955 study of cervical dilation in laboring women. Friedman plotted the labors of five hundred women on a graph to determine how long it took each woman's cervix to open wide enough for her baby to be born. He found that active labor began when a woman's cervix dilated four centimeters. Once active labor was underway, birth attendants could expect an average cervical dilation of three centimeters per hour, until the cervix was dilated nine centimeters. Less dilation than the three centimeters per hour that Friedman predicted was thereafter seen as abnormal and meant that something was wrong. The rate of normal antici- pated dilation is called the Friedman curve. It became the basis for measuring labor length and progress in hospitals and helped cement guidelines for when to operate if someone's labor appears to have stalled.

But many say the data are problematic. Friedman's five hundred subjects were all white and gave birth in the same hospital. About 13 percent of them were induced with Pitocin, more than half of deliver- ies were assisted by forceps, and a whopping 96 percent of the birthers were sedated. In other words, what has become standard labor length for all people was based on what seems to be a flawed study of the hos- pital labor of white women in the 1950s altered by tools and drugs. Yet the Friedman curve is somehow still presented in textbooks and taught in medical schools—where, remember, obstetrical dilemma thinking thrives.

As Rebecca Dekker, founder of Evidence Based Birth, told me, we really can't apply old data to people who birth today. "In Dr. Fried- man's time, if you were dilating at about one centimeter per hour, that was too slow," she said. "You would be considered to have failure to progress or abnormal labor. Today, research is finding very different averages for what is normal."

For instance, newer studies have discovered that active labor be- gins when a woman's cervix has dilated to six, not four, centimeters. Meaning that it can take more time to reach active labor. Researchers have now shown that three centimeters per hour was abnormally fast for dilation. One centimeter per hour is more standard, meaning the average labor takes far *longer* than Friedman thought.

Looking at nearly 230,000 birth records, Jun Zhang and his col- leagues found that half of all C-sections performed for dystocia, or "failure to progress," after labor induction came before pregnant peo- ple had even reached six centimeters dilation. To reduce unnecessary C-sections, the researchers advised that "cesarean section for dystocia should be avoided before the active phase is established." Put simply, don't cut people open before their labor even begins.

Although modern studies have established that normal labor likely takes longer, they are not without limitations and biases either, because of how and where the births took place. More than 40 percent of the births Zhang studied were induced with Pitocin, and 90 percent involved epidurals. These interventions alter how labor occurs and its duration. Shockingly, I am aware of no large-scale studies of physiologic labor—looking only at people who birth without intervention—to determine a standard of labor. Until such a study is conducted, women must contend with the status quo: if you give birth in a hospital, your body and labor must adhere to standards established by problematic studies of birth interventions. And if those standards aren't met—say, because you refuse Pitocin and your labor is taking longer than "normal"—you will be encouraged, and perhaps eventually forced, to have a C-section.

Friedman doesn't practice anymore—he's in his nineties. Wayne Cohen, a former chief of obstetrics at Jacobi Medical Center in the Bronx, trained as a resident under Friedman. Cohen told me that both he and Friedman take issue with the newer curves found by Zhang and others. He said that Friedman's research has been misinterpreted— that the lower limit of the curve that Friedman found was 1.2 centimeters dilation per hour and that 3 centimeters dilation per hour was "never used in clinical guidelines." In short, Friedman didn't actually underestimate how long labor takes.

Cohen and Friedman have publicly challenged assertions that Friedman's curve is flawed. They point out in a 2020 essay in the *American Journal of Obstetrics and Gynecology* that, despite the adoption of new labor curve guidelines, "there has been no major fall in caesarean delivery frequency." In fact, they note that while the cesarean rate quadrupled between 1970 and 2000, when Friedman's curve was predominantly in use, the application of the newer labor curve hasn't thus far reduced the cesarean rate. They believe that other factors must be at work, doubling down on their curve results and questioning the math of the newer curves. They are correct that physicians' schedules, hospitals' risk intolerance, fear of litigation, and moneymaking all fuel cesareans. But citing "relevant demographic changes in the pregnant population" and concerns about patient choice raising the rate misses the mark. We know elective C-sections account for only around 2 to 3 percent of the total. And to propose that diet, age, and underlying health conditions are causing more C-sections, as Cohen and Friedman do, is to blame women instead of doctors and hospitals.

Maybe the problem is applying curves in hospitals. Consider the difference between hospital births and home births. In hospitals, "failure to progress" remains the top reason for C-sections in the United States today. And, overall, C-sections constitute about 35 percent of all births. With home births, in contrast, "failure to progress" is only diagnosed 4 percent of the time. In other words, where physiologic labors are supported, encouraged, and allowed to unfold without timers, pressure, and protocols, labor progresses normally 96 percent of the time. Perhaps it's birth location, not "failure to progress," that causes unnecessary C-sections. Or, as Julienne Rutherford, Kylea Liese, and Ifeyinwa Asidou put it in the *American Journal of Human Biology*, "As currently deployed, the concept of 'failure to progress' is anchored in fault, and the locus of that fault lies explicitly within the machinery of the human body of the laboring person that is escaping management."

I WAS LABORING WITH MY SECOND CHILD IN THE HOSPITAL WHEN a nurse entered the room and asked me to get onto a table.

I'd rather stand, I said.

Put this on, she said.

The electronic fetal monitor is a little box attached to elastic bands that are strapped around the belly. From the box extends a cord that's plugged into a monitoring machine on a stand with a display screen— the kind common throughout hospitals, which you've likely seen if you've been to an emergency room. The contraption tracks the baby's heart rate alongside the duration and frequency of the mom's contractions. If the baby is exhibiting "nonreassuring fetal heart tones"—a broad, murky category—hospital staff fear that the baby isn't tolerating labor well, and C-section can be ordered.

Hospitals prefer to monitor laborers continuously and remotely, not intermittently and in person. The former is less work for staff, and ideal when fewer doctors and nurses are at work; they can supervise multiple people at once remotely from the nurses' station. Laborers who are monitored intermittently alternate between wearing and removing the band, sometimes for hours or even days. LaToya did this with the help of her doula to go to the bathroom. Continuous monitoring confines people to beds where providers can easily access their abdomens. They're told to lie still so that the machine's tracing isn't compromised. Those stretchy bands are less likely to slip off a stationary belly than a moving one. Restricted movement during labor, like being stuck on your back or seated on a table for monitoring, can be uncomfortable and cause labor to stall. Those positions make things easier for doctors and nurses, not for women.

The nurse allowed me to stand, then stretched a double band around my tightening stomach. Wanting to be a good patient, I acquiesced. She didn't introduce herself, explain monitoring, ask my permission, make a recommendation, or tell me her purpose. She just did it and then walked out. My tracings were now available at the nurses' station. After she left, I still didn't know what the bands were, what I had been hooked to. It was safe to say that mentally I was inside my body, which was a completely different place from inside that room. My animal brain was fighting with my manners and logic.

Oh, this is a … monitor, I finally said, momentarily failing to remember its full name. It was jarring to be laboring in a bright room and also to be expected to respond to those who were speaking to me. Talking during a contraction was becoming impossible. I watched the screen through one, curious about what the wavy lines would do. They lifted and lowered. OK, so that's what that's like, I thought. Quickly I forgot about it, back in my body again, down in the enveloping dark. I began to walk, widening my gait and swaying my hips a little, as if a song I liked had come on. But as I moved, I felt a tug at my middle. I lurched forward but was then snapped back, pinned in place by the leash. Frustrated, I loosened the tether so I could move. The nurse returned—she had probably heard the alarm squeal, indicating that

my contractions and my baby's heart tones weren't being detected—
and asked what was going on. Why wasn't I wearing the monitor? I
couldn't form my desire not to wear it into a sentence. And then another contraction began.

Can she labor without it for now? my doula asked, so kind. Yes, exactly, I thought, but that idea was choked by an internal current pulsing
through my stomach and limbs. I spread my legs in a plié, feet gripping
the ground. I opened my lips and throat and let out a long, low sound.
I pinched my eyes shut, then relaxed the lids. A red and blue pattern
emerged on the backs of them. I was moving as if a ghost had whirled
through my body. As my contraction subsided, my anger flared.

I'm pretty sure I already declined fetal monitoring in my birth plan,
but I'd like to decline it again, I said, petulantly. The nurse gave me
a look, meant both to shame and convey skepticism. Or maybe surprise? Then, she left.

If you've had a baby in a hospital, you were almost certainly hooked
up to an electronic fetal monitor. If you weren't attached, either you
arrived at the hospital with a crowning baby, or you are a delivery
room Houdini. Monitoring is practically mandatory in hospitals. The
Listening to Mothers surveyors found about 90 percent of people who
labored in hospitals were surveilled. More than half were monitored
continuously, meaning that the wearers couldn't move freely. A re-
straint bound them to a machine.

The monitor, a combination ultrasound device and pressure sen-
sor, is perhaps the most ubiquitous technology in all of childbirth.
It tracks three things: the baby's heart rate and the laboring person's
contraction length and frequency, which appear as line graphs on
a screen, called tracings. Sensors detect a baby's baseline heart rate
(interchangeable here with tone) and how it changes during contractions. An increase in heart rate is called acceleration; a decrease, de-
celeration. The change in the rate is called a fetal heart tracing. Birth
attendants periodically review the fetal heart tracings, they say, to understand whether labor is going well.

You can be monitored internally and externally. External monitoring is more common. That's the pair of belts wrapped around your

middle. Internal monitoring can only happen after membranes have ruptured, meaning your water has broken. In that case, electrodes are inserted into the vagina and cervix and attached to baby's scalp (or other presenting part) to measure their heart rate. It's *very* invasive. In birth, it's preferable for things to exit the vagina, not the other way around.

Electronic fetal monitors are the second leading cause of unnecessary C-sections. They are presented as a labor necessity when they can cause untold harm. How they evolved to attach to nearly every birthing person and why they remain there today is a maddening story.

Edward Hon, a postdoctoral fellow at Yale, discovered in 1958 that continuously measuring the fetal heartbeat during labor could determine whether the baby was in distress. His finding helped create the first commercial monitor in 1968. By 1970, monitors had hit hospital delivery units, promising to prevent cerebral palsy—a movement disorder linked to abnormal brain development or damage—by detecting a baby's real-time stress level. Doctors once assumed that birth asphyxia commonly caused cerebral palsy and believed monitors could stop it.

Simultaneously, medical malpractice lawsuits exploded in the 1960s, accelerating an insurance coverage crisis for doctors and hospitals in the 1970s. Obstetrics was targeted because "the only evidence of fetal heart rate during labor had been the obstetrician's recollection." That is, until electronic fetal monitoring (EFM) arrived, wrote Thomas Sartwelle, James Johnston, and Berna Arda, a lawyer, neurologist, and medical ethicist, respectively, in a riveting 2017 essay about the flaws of monitoring. Trial lawyers used electronic fetal monitors "to extract billions from physicians and hospitals the world over" by bringing monitor tracings to court to show "the precise moment the inattentive or ignorant physician should have performed a C-section to save what courtroom experts said was a neurologically perfect infant from lifelong crippling injuries." But soon, doctors and hospitals retaliated, using electronic fetal monitoring in the same way the trial lawyers did—as a defensive measure deployed to protect themselves, not mothers and babies. Unnecessary and risky interventions have increased ever since, C-sections chief among them. Monitoring "remains immune to the doctrine of informed consent despite continually mounting evidence which proves the procedure is nothing more than myth, illusion and junk science that subjects mothers and babies alike to increased risks of morbidity and mortality," Sartwelle, Johnston, and Arda conclude. They call present monitoring use "an egregious conflict of interest and outrageous endorsement of obstetrical defensive medicine" and "the epitome of medical paternalism."

We assume that new technology is first robustly studied and scrutinized by scientists, experts, and governments before being assimilated into hospitals for near total use. Instead, monitors were cleverly marketed—first by creating a fear of a rare pediatric condition, cerebral palsy, and then by selling a supposed prophylactic. Evidence about the effectiveness and safety of monitoring technology was gathered only from the women who were first subjected to it in the 1970s—those who found themselves in hospitals to which monitor hawkers were marketing. But staff didn't tell them that the monitors weren't supported by medical evidence. They didn't even tell them what they were. Women were simply told, just like I was nearly fifty years later, to put it on. "It's a common pattern that women are guinea pigs," Dekker of Evidence Based Birth told me. "Instead of studying it first, let's just do it to everybody."

Monitors do not do what the manufacturers and medical establishment initially promised they would do. Cerebral palsy develops in utero or infancy, rarely if ever as the result of labor and delivery. Rates of the condition haven't changed much since monitoring's advent. It's a similar story for other adverse labor and delivery outcomes. Randomized controlled trials show that electronic fetal monitoring doesn't improve rates of stillbirth or newborn death, brain damage, NICU admission, or other birth complications. The authors of the second edition of *Neonatal Encephalopathy and Neurologic Outcome*, a 2014 publication from ACOG and the American Academy of Pediatrics, conceded that "there is no evidence to predict neonatal neurologic injury, cerebral palsy, or stillbirth using Electronic Fetal

Monitoring" and that "cesarean delivery as an obstetrical intervention to reduce neonatal encephalopathy and cerebral palsy has been considered unsuccessful." They found that monitoring offers "no long-term benefits as currently used."

No benefits, just harms, yet monitors remain commonplace. Obstetricians have likened their use to an addiction. They can observe multiple labors at once without being present or providing an ounce of support. Practically speaking, birth wards are busy places, and monitors can feel like an extra pair of hands. One of the monitor's developers, Orvan Hess, also an early adopter of penicillin use, believed tracking fetal distress would eliminate the "watch and wait and pray" theme in childbirth. Before monitoring, "the uterus was literally a black box," obstetrician Joshua Copel said. "We knew the babies were in there, and they came out." Today, an electronic monitor is strapped to or inserted inside the bodies of millions of laboring people, not because the technology has proven helpful, but because doctors want to see inside at every moment. Even if the device's information is opaque.

"The tool itself does what it does, it tells you what the baby's heart rate is," Aaron Caughey, chief of obstetrics and gynecology at Oregon Health Sciences University, told NPR in 2014. "But there's a problem on the interpretation side of things, trying to determine what the changes of the fetal heart rate really mean. We don't really understand the tool all that well." Doctors trust a gadget that seems to provide practically useless information instead of the woman before them.

Hospitals won't dispense with electronic fetal monitors for two reasons that have nothing to do with the well-being of birthing people: liability and profit. Electronic fetal monitors create a record of what staff did during a birth, which is still desirable when hospitals face lawsuits. They also represent massive investment. One survey found that there are twenty-eight thousand monitors in more than thirty-four hundred US hospitals—which cost more than $700 million to purchase. Though most hospitals can't collect separate insurance claims for routine monitoring, the cost of monitoring has helped elevate the total cost of hospital birth. And internal monitoring or monitoring done by a specialist can produce a separate insurance charge for birthers. The global fetal monitoring analysis market—which includes devices such as ultrasound and electronic fetal monitors—is growing. It was estimated at $3.7 billion in 2021 and expected to reach $5.2 billion by 2026.

It's hard to escape the visual and the feeling of what monitoring is. A tether, a leash. It prevents movement, pins you in place. It sends data to a computer. White coats in another room watch your body function, your baby's pumping blood. It's dystopian. Especially when, as Sartwelle, Johnston, and Arda put it, "EFM as a screening tool for absence of harm is no better than tossing a coin."

The second leading cause of C-sections, essentially monitoring, can even cause the first, Dekker explains. Because if you're laboring in place, unable to move, it can halt labor and cause "failure to progress." "Hooking someone up to an electronic fetal monitor increases risks to the mother without significantly improving safety for the baby," she says. And doctors will tell you they like it because they can keep an eye on you. And when they have the monitor to watch, they can tune into it instead of you.

INCREASINGLY, WE'RE LEARNING WHAT OUR ANCESTORS KNEW— we need labor support, not surveillance. More touch, fewer tools.

Monitoring laboring people with a gizmo that hasn't been tested and that we now know causes harm has nudged out a perfectly good practice: intermittent auscultation, or hands-on listening. This was used during all of my pregnancies, beginning with prenatal visits. There are different devices for this method of assessing the baby's condition during pregnancy and labor. Hospital midwives used a handheld Doppler to detect the fetal heartbeat using sound waves. My home birth midwife carried a fetoscope, essentially a stethoscope designed for uteruses. Another type is called a pinard, which is small and horn shaped. The beauty and effectiveness of the hands-on technique is that it also necessitates physical touch. The midwife places her hands on your body. She palpates your abdomen. She might look into your eyes. It's intimate.

I would climb up onto the table in the midwife's office, and she would apply the Doppler, gliding the flat top of the wand over my gel-coated abdomen. At home, I laid on my couch, and the midwife put the end of what looked like a stethoscope on my belly. She would sate the curiosity of my other children by allowing them to also move one end around to different parts of my increasingly round stomach. Then she would hand them earpieces the size of quarters so they could listen to the *pwah pwah* of their future sibling's heart. It was easily the best part of my week.

Intermittent auscultation can be used to track a baby's heart rate in most laboring people. However, it's nearly impossible to find intermittent auscultation in US hospitals. Nurses, doctors, and even midwives practicing in medical settings rarely do it. Most of them don't know how. Intermittent auscultation requires training. You have to be able to locate the baby's heart while using the senses of sound and touch. It takes time. The sound can be hard to pinpoint, as babies move during pregnancy, and there are many other sounds to hear. You must also be able to distinguish between a baby's heartbeat and the mom's, as both sounds can filter into the earpiece. With training, you can even hear a baby's heartbeat with a toilet paper tube. During labor, a provider can use a Doppler or a fetal stethoscope to listen at intervals, which is far less invasive than constantly wearing an electronic fetal monitor around your middle or having one inserted into your vagina as you're working to push your baby out. Handheld Dopplers are cheaper technology too; they run between $400 and $500, whereas monitoring systems cost around $20,000 each. During my home birth, my midwife listened with her Doppler to my abdomen once. That was it.

Hands-on listening is the safest and most evidence-supported method for hearing the fetal heartbeat in most pregnant people. To start, it produces fewer birth interventions—fewer C-sections, fewer forceps and vacuum deliveries. A 2017 review of the literature by the Cochrane Pregnancy and Childbirth database, comparing hands-on listening to electronic fetal monitoring, revealed that people who were monitored continuously were 63 percent more likely to have a C-section and 15 percent more likely to birth with vacuum or forceps than those who experienced hands-on listening in their births. Intermittent auscultation is also linked to more and better labor support for women. The Doppler or fetal stethoscope allows for movement in labor. The equipment is far less expensive and easier to maintain. Yet, despite these benefits, the method is dying out. Only about 11 percent of births use it today.

In EFM, an electronic fetal monitor is strapped on, and that's that. Intermittent auscultation requires more effort. The procedure is recommended about every half hour during labor. This means a trained practitioner can't watch the wiggly tracing lines from another room, alongside the wiggly lines of half a dozen other people. She must be with the laboring person, touching her body, using the fetoscope, Doppler, or pinard.

The resistance to the simpler technology can manifest in nefarious ways. I heard a story about a laboring woman transferring to a hospital with her midwife and partner. The emergency medicine technicians openly mocked the midwife for doing hands-on listening. Birth environments that disparage or resist hands-on listening tend to shirk in-person labor support and disregard what those giving birth actually need and want.

"If hospitals were willing to invest in more hands-on care to support women during childbirth, we would likely see more hands-on listening," Dekker wrote. We would also see fewer C-sections, less use of forceps and vacuum extraction, and likely fewer traumatic births.

Friedman and Cohen are right about one thing: the use of the Friedman curve is not the only thing causing unnecessary operations. What must be examined is the dysfunctional relationship dynamics hospitals foster between physicians and their pregnant patients: a lack of trust, trepidation about litigation, prioritization of profit, and the deliberate creation of fear as a means of controlling women.

If women's bodies are naturally suspect and irrevocably flawed, it makes sense to limit the amount of time they are permitted to labor and, when their time is up, to cut them off and slice them open. If obstetrics believes its job is to control childbirth, manage labor with tools, and perform surgery, if pregnant bodies seem incapable to them, or in need of rescue, then C-section rates will remain high or climb. Millions of people will continue to experience birth trauma and postpartum pain and complications. Too many will continue to suffer, and too many will die.

LISBETH REMEMBERS BEING UNDERDRESSED FOR HOW COLD THE room was after having traded her clothes for a stiff cap and blue gown. Maria waited for thirteen hours. Nurses forbade eating, and she struggled to breathe, recalling the time as a long, slow panic attack. Lying on the operating table, Gwen felt cocooned, as if she were alone in a camping tent. She couldn't see the surgeon, only the cone of fabric enclosing her. LaToya remembers the oxygen mask pressed to her face, occluding her vision, and the shock of being strapped down, then the stupor. Her arms and wrists were glued to the table. Nearly all the women I've talked to about their C-sections recount this detail—being chained to the table—how powerless and abused they felt, how no one told them about that part before it happened or explained why when it did. LaToya described it as being bound, like on a cross. Another mother felt trapped like an animal.

When C-sections are ordered, women submit to measures that transform them from person to patient. This process is marked by discomfort and fear. You're stripped down, metaphorically and actually. Some protocols are designed for safety. Others are holdover traditions based in eminence, not evidence. Many are intrinsically inhumane, but their purported necessity goes unexplained. Strapping down birthers isn't compulsory for C-section safety, nor is it universal. It's more a means to protect doctors from patients jostling them than to benefit those being operated on.

To add insult to injury (or gaslighting to trauma), those who birth surgically later often find themselves in the position of defending C-section as a valid form of birth, rather than a failure of the medical establishment, internalizing the idea that the turn of events was their own fault. They buy into the prevailing myth that real womanhood, pure motherhood, is only achievable through natural, vaginal birth.

This lie requires C-section mothers to justify how they delivered, even if the way they delivered wasn't their choice, but due to actual medical necessity or, more likely, to convenience and coercion. One woman told me her C-section made her question "whether or not I could claim I was a real mom." I have talked to others who felt that, because they didn't push, they were deprived of a "real birth."

"I still feel like a total failure because my body did not behave the way it was supposed to, and my deliveries do not feel like something I successfully did but rather something that was done to me because I wasn't capable enough to manage on my own," said Amber, who experienced two C-sections in rural Mississippi, both after preeclampsia diagnoses.

Imposter syndrome—doubt in oneself and fear of being exposed as a fraud—plagues women and Black, Brown, trans, and nonbinary people in many areas of life, including childbirth. I've heard the term C-section imposter syndrome used in birth-work circles to describe the outcropping of forces beyond the control of individual birthing people. Birthers are made to feel guilty for feeling anything but gratitude for what they have been told was a lifesaving procedure. Any other relationship described this way would be deemed abusive. But not the one between a mother and her doctor, at least not by most people. C-section imposter syndrome causes birthers to blame themselves and their bodies instead of the well-oiled medical system, which operates on women unnecessarily all the time.

Another piece of so-called C-section imposter syndrome is that no one acknowledges the shock and suffering that result when a birth plan goes awry. More often, birthers are shamed for making a birth plan. They're told not to bother preparing for labor, because in labor nothing goes to plan. They're mocked for trying to orchestrate the perfect birth, as if it were a beautiful but hollow thing, an Instagram post. They're made to relinquish control. If not explicitly, then passive aggressively, with tacit eye rolls, sighs, diminutives.

LaToya blamed the surgery for the challenges she faced as a new mother. When she struggled to breastfeed right away, she held the operation responsible—it had caused nurses to give her baby formula and to separate her from her infant for too long.

"You know, if she got a diaper rash—and she did get bad diaper rash—I'm like, 'Oh it's because I had a C-section,'" LaToya told me. She felt her daughter had missed out on the beneficial vaginal bacteria she would have been exposed to during birth—that was why her diaper rash was so inflamed. LaToya blamed the C-section for why she didn't get enough time with her newborn before returning to work—there was more healing for her body to do than she had anticipated, which interrupted bonding. The baby's low iron? Need for eyedrops? C-section. "We didn't get started on the right foot, my baby and I," she said. "It's not true but that's what was true for me in my head. I'm like, 'This is because of this C-section. These things are happening because of this.'"

When the surgeons were stitching LaToya up, she saw a flash of green in her peripheral vision. "One of the doctors is near my head, and he has a menu," she recalled. "I think the menu is laminated. They're talking about what they're going to order for dinner. After this surgery. 'Do you feel like Chinese? Or a diner?' They're talking about food. This is a day at work for them. They should think more about what they're talking about when they have a patient on the table. They're delivering that person's child, and it's a major moment in your life. I'm never going to forget the fact that they were talking about what to eat."

LaToya refers to herself in the second person, distancing herself from the trauma. Most of the birth was fuzzy. She wasn't the first person to hold the baby. Her midwife and husband held her daughter before she did. When LaToya finally saw her child, she was wrapped in a blanket and wearing a hat.

"After that surgery, I felt like I wasn't put back together the same. Emotionally and physically I just wasn't the same person after that experience," LaToya told me.

IN THE LATE 2000s, BETH ISRAEL DEACONESS MEDICAL CENTER in Brookline, Massachusetts, had one of the highest C-section rates in the country, said Toni Golen, vice chair of obstetrics and gynecology

at the hospital, when I interviewed her. "We decided that was something we wanted to decrease and that it was important," she said. The
hospital has since cut its C-section rate by half in a little more than a
decade.

Golen said that since the 1950s the hospital had used the Friedman
curve to define whether a labor was progressing at a standard pace.
What they started to realize was that to improve birth and reduce
the cesarean delivery rate, they needed to improve their diagnosis of
stalled labor. "Labor is not a one-size-fits-all proposition," she said.
"Every person can have a different labor and just because it might be
different from a person in the room next door doesn't mean that it's
abnormal."

Golen and her team made a change. Instead of interpreting active
labor as beginning at four centimeters, as Friedman had directed,
they began to use Zhang's six centimeters. "There's a conversation that
happens among the nurse, the resident physician, the attending physician, the midwife, and we typically will tell the story of how a labor
is progressing," Golen explained. Leading that conversation, Golen
said, is the question, "Is the patient in the active phase or not?" Golen
elaborated, "If you make the decision that the patient is in the active
phase, then you have a certain expectation for cervical change. If the
patient fails that and that doesn't happen, then it opens the door to
make the decision to recommend a cesarean delivery."

The newer data about when active labor begins shifted the Boston
hospital's approach: "That conversation changed as a result of endors-
ing the Zhang data, and it changed in really concrete ways. Everyone
adhered to the practice that we couldn't really apply the rules of what
we would expect cervical change to be at four centimeters. We had
to wait until six centimeters. I would say that was the single most important thing."

The labor and delivery unit also began offering "supportive care,"
which means allowing people more time to labor and discussing their
options with them rather than simply imposing protocol—especially
when mediations and anesthesia are involved. But in addition, "supportive care" also includes introducing and committing to low-tech

options: suggesting that the birthing person might be able to ease the labor by changing positions, moving around, trying a birthing ball, or receiving massage, which can encourage relaxation. The other notable action Golen and her colleagues took was centering laboring women and acknowledging that they are the experts in their own bodies. It's a strategy as old as labor itself, but in the modern sense, it's borrowed from the midwifery model of care.

Lastly, Beth Israel Deaconess is scrupulous with metrics. They calculate their total cesarean delivery rate and the rate for first-time moms, since Golen knows that reducing these C-sections is crucial to lowering the overall rate. They also measure the C-section rates of individual doctors and share them at department meetings, during rounds, and even on social media. "We've created a little bit of healthy competition around it," Golen said. "We praise publicly and criticize in private."

Three thousand miles from greater Boston, Overlake Medical Center in Bellevue, Washington, delivers about thirty-three hundred babies each year with a staff of seventy-five labor and delivery nurses and around sixty obstetricians and midwives. Margie Bridges, a nurse there for more than two decades, called Overlake's C-section rate, which has toggled between 30 and 40 percent, "one of the best of the worst." "It's not for lack of effort," she added.

Overlake had tried many of the same strategies as Beth Israel, but without success, Bridges shared. Even though it tossed the Friedman curve, offered support measures, and set tangible goals, Overlake's rate had been stuck at around 30 percent for six years. They had also reduced the rate of inductions and delayed admitting pregnant women until they were an active six centimeters, a practice that guidelines suggest can lessen the chances of C-sections. The struggle came to a head when an insurance company took notice of the high rate and demanded that the hospital decrease the number of expensive surgeries they were billing for. "It was like, 'What else can we do?'" Bridges recalls asking. "We've really struggled."

So Overlake attempted something simple that turned out to be radical—an old tool used in a new way. They took large white dry erase boards, like the kind you would buy at a home goods store, and put one in each labor and delivery room. Anyone can write on it, but the board must contain a number of things. On it go the names of the birthing person and her partner, along with her core team: doctor, doula, midwife, anesthesiologist, and so forth. Next are the birthing person's labor preferences, such as wanting the ability to move around during active labor, or to decline an electronic fetal monitor. These preferences aren't fixed; they can change if a laboring person decides they should. Next, the status of the mom, the baby (how they are doing), and labor progress are included. Lastly, the time the entire birth team (everyone whose names are on the board) will convene next is listed. This helps ensure that all of the conversations taking place about a particular woman and her labor are occurring with her present, not at the remote nurses' station or without key people in the room. Bridges likened typical communication between a care team during labor to a game of telephone, where the original message gets lost by the time it is passed around. That's what Overlake is trying to prevent.

"It gets very muddled in labor as far as what we're doing sometimes," Bridges told me. But the white board has changed that. It centers the laboring person and her desires and needs. It has the benefit of clarifying each step in a woman's birth story. She's aware of what's going on, and she's part of the decision-making at every turn.

Overlake's rate is declining. In 2020, the hospital recorded a 26 percent C-section rate in first-time deliveries. That's still higher than the hospital would like, but it's trending in the right direction. I wonder what it would take to close that gap, for these collaborations to produce a better understanding of how to lower C-section rates and support women.

Evergreen Health in Kirkland, Washington, is another facility using the white boards and team huddles for births and studying the results. That's where Kelsey Mooseker gave birth to her twins.

"The white board was an amazing planning tool," she told me, just days after delivering, from Evergreen hospital, where she was working on breastfeeding her twins and preparing to bring them home.

Kelsey had known that she didn't want to push on her back. Her OB, Bettina Paek, wrote that down on the white board. She also wanted her doula and husband with her. Paek wrote that down too. Her birth team knew her history and incorporated it into her chart. During that first labor and birth, she "really felt like everything was being done to me," she said. "Now, it was like, 'What do you want?' To be asked that question as a laboring mom is powerful and it gives you the power to say what you want and to be heard. It made me feel like I was being heard." Bridges, at Overlake, said that the white board is almost unanimously appreciated in the surveys they collect from new moms.

The white board and huddle design don't "address all of the systemic factors that may be affecting safety and dignity of childbirth care across the United States, such as limited prenatal education or explicit bias," the white board program creators at Harvard's Ariadne Labs wrote in an article summarizing their findings in the journal *Birth*. But as for designing a care plan "that aims to improve communication and teamwork between clinicians and patients" in hospitals, this is a promising start.

The tactics hospitals are using to reduce C-sections look an awful lot like birth before it was medicalized. At the turn of the twentieth century, remember, most people gave birth at home surrounded by women—a midwife attendant with birth expertise along with family members and friends. Social childbirth centered the birther. What's now called the Midwives Model of Care maintains that pregnancy and childbirth are "normal life events," as the Midwives Alliance of North America puts it, not a sickness or disorder. Midwifery's core characteristics are "being with women, listening to women, and sharing knowledge and decision-making with women." Avoiding unnecessary technological intervention is critical.

Doula support also reduces C-sections. Typically, doulas are hired by pregnant people to be with them and advocate for their needs during birth. There are more than twenty-three hundred doulas in the registry of DONA International, the organization that trains and certifies the most doulas in the US. Doulas now play the role once occupied by friends and family in the days of social childbirth. In one of the best studies of doulas, researchers assigned 420 first-time moms to either partner support or both doula and partner support during labor. Researchers found that 13 percent of the moms with partner and doula support had C-sections, while 25 percent of those with only partner support did. Doula presence alone reduced C-sections by half.

MY FRIEND LISBETH, A CHILDREN'S BOOK AUTHOR, OFFERED TO tell me about her gentle C-section, a procedure I'd never heard of before she mentioned it to me on the sidewalk one day after our postpartum exercise class. I wanted to know more, so we got coffee. I put down my bag and tape recorder. Two other moms I knew roosted at a neighboring table.

Lisbeth told me that her first C-section was both unexpected and unwanted. She had desired and planned for a vaginal birth without intervention. In the hypnobirthing class Lisbeth hosted in her home, the instructor treated C-section like a curse. She had refused to say the word, as if doing so would cast it into being. But after Lisbeth had labored for eight hours and pushed to the point of crowning, her midwife recommended the operation, and Lisbeth, suffering and exhausted, agreed.

Awaiting surgery felt like readying "for the guillotine," she said. She remembers a rude resident who shook and tugged her, which "felt like he was enacting violence." After her daughter was born, Lisbeth hemorrhaged and struggled to remain conscious during the blood loss. Her husband, Alex, watched the surgery and his wife in a panic, which later caused him post-traumatic stress disorder.

"He was worried that I was going to die," Lisbeth said. "And I was just focusing on not dying, which is a very different experience." Once she was stable, Lisbeth turned her attention to her infant. She didn't want to dwell on her birth.

A few years later, when Lisbeth and her doctor chose a C-section because her second baby was in a breech position, she wanted it to go differently. Her obstetrician told her about the option of a "gentle C-section"—a different approach to the traditional surgery. However, he warned that the procedure wasn't always permitted in the hospital where they would deliver. They might have to do it "on the sly," or they might be prevented from doing it at all. He said that he wouldn't know until the day of her scheduled surgery. "Some nurses and support staff will help with this, and some are hard liners and won't," he told her. "So, we'll do our best to make this a gentle C-section," even though, as Lisbeth put it, "the hospital wasn't on board."

In the end, Lisbeth lucked out. The operation took place slowly, with one obstetrician standing by her head, another posted at her midsection, explaining to Lisbeth and Alex what they were doing in real time. Her obstetrician lowered the drape that hung above her torso so that they could witness their daughter being lifted up out of her belly, being born. He swabbed the newborn with a cloth of vaginal secretions, which he had pocketed, to give her body and immune system the benefits of the birth canal. He placed the infant on Lisbeth's chest so they could bond skin-to-skin and delayed what could wait—the Apgar test, vitamin K administration, weight and height measurements.

Before the surgery, Lisbeth's obstetrician had instructed her to tie the strings of her hospital gown around the back of her neck like a halter top, so that she could tug on one string and let the fabric fall away to breastfeed, which she did. "But he was like, 'Don't show this to anyone! And I don't know if it does anything,' but I just loved that there was somebody working for me. Trying to help."

Women described their C-sections to me with words like "dehumanizing," "sterile," "terrifying," "violent," and "cold." Lisbeth's birth is proof that it doesn't need to be this way.

I've since heard what she experienced called "gentle," "natural," "family-friendly," or "family-centered C-section." It aims to give women all the beauty and wonder of birth. It's both a new style of caregiving, of operating, and a mindset. Gentle C-sections don't dispense with the rules meant to protect people in surgery. They work to lessen their limitations. And unlike during her first surgery, this time Lisbeth knew exactly what was happening.

Midwife Jenny Smith helped create the practice. She describes the hallmarks of gentle C-sections in the 2008 journal article "The Natural Caesarean: A Woman-Centered Technique." Smith recommends that birthers and their partners meet with the surgeon and ideally visit the operating theater ahead of the scheduled date. But that's almost never done.

Smith lists technical changes to the procedure that allow women to see the birth if they wish and to hold their babies immediately after. The amount of anesthesia is important—sufficient for pain prevention but not enough to impair the mother. She needs free hands for baby holding, thus the pulse oximeter, which measures oxygen in red blood cells, should be clipped to her toe rather than her finger. The intravenous line for fluids should sit in the nondominant arm, and the electrocardiogram measuring her heart rate should be placed away from the chest wall. The drape is lowered for the birth, as was the case for Lisbeth. Some hospitals offer a clear drape, so birthers and partners can watch the birth through the sterile screen. Smith found that those who have gentle C-sections embraced them with "no adverse comment in more than 100 procedures." Lisbeth described her gentle C-section as a "healing birth." "I realized that I had a beautiful C-section. How many people can say that?" she said.

Gentle C-section isn't a common offering. Most people don't know to ask for it. Others are refused. When Rachel asked for a gentle C-section in New York City, her doctors balked. "My concerns were brushed off as not relevant," she said. "And my wishes for a kinder, gentler C-section were dismissed as not possible during this medical procedure." Amber said being denied a more humane C-section contributed to her postpartum depression and anxiety. "Despite my ardent requests, I didn't even get to do immediate skin-to-skin with my newborn because we were at a rural hospital in Mississippi and they weren't set up for that."

Why aren't gentle C-sections being offered everywhere? Smith believes the barrier isn't something meaningful, like safety or even cost—she and her colleagues found no difference. The barrier mirrors the reason there are too many C-sections to begin with: a system's stubborn refusal to change. But change is possible. There's a ready blueprint. For some, it's happening right now.

Ultimately, Lisbeth's gentle C-section was healing not only because her care team was willing to help her achieve a more humane, personal experience but because she decided to center herself in her birth, to be the most important person in the room.

"My OBs helped me in every way to have those moments that I wanted that are so beautiful from birth. I mentally imagined being in control of this. And I was."

CHAPTER 7
CONSENTING YOU

I call my second labor the long one. Unlike my speedy maiden birth, it allowed me to slow down and experience the process. My contractions were steady and manageable most of the time, and my water didn't break until the very end. Since there was no rush, I knew better than to haul ass to the hospital. That morning, I had sex with my husband (in an attempt to start labor; it worked), I read a book, I dressed my daughter and took her out to play with her grandparents. I strolled down Court Street with my brother, pausing to grasp scaffolding when a contraction hit, doubled over labyrinthine bars. At home I made nachos—dicing tomatoes, sprinkling cheese, dislodging pickled jalapeños from a jar—and ate standing up. As the contractions came and went, I was happy to be at home. And since there wasn't a crowning head, I didn't see why I couldn't be.

As the day waned, the breaks between contractions shortened. I was undoubtedly in active labor. Ben wondered if maybe we should just go already. Remember how fast it happened last time? he asked. And how making it to the hospital was my fear? Begrudgingly, I packed a bag, believing this was premature. My dad drove us to the hospital. I spent the ride complaining that we were arriving too soon. Sarah, our doula, met us in the waiting room outside triage. I lumbered in circles, pausing to lean on the wall.

More than an hour later, a nurse with dark cropped hair and a long face invited me into a pantry-sized exam room. She didn't ask whether or not I wanted to be examined. She handed me a cotton gown and told me to put it on. At the time, this felt completely normal: I would remove my clothes and allow a nurse to plunge her hand into my vagina sans explanation. I had heard that the finger metric to assess dilation would determine whether I'd be admitted to the hospital.

I *wanted* to be admitted. I wanted to meet my kid. I didn't want the nurse to send me home. Therefore, I needed to offer my vagina to gloved fingers, in the midst of rippling contractions. Hospital admission would only be possible if preceded by a vaginal exam yielding the correct information. So I didn't ask the nurse why she was conducting a vaginal exam, and I didn't stop her. I thought that I wanted her to do it. I wanted to breach the gate. I didn't want to creep around the lobby anymore, leaning on stuff. The procedure didn't seem optional. It wasn't explained at all.

The nurse consented me, a term that I didn't know then but have learned since. It's when providers make a patient say yes to something, like a procedure or drug. Stating a choice as a fact—"We're going to examine you now"—is one of many methods. This nurse in the teddy bear scrubs consented me. I'd wager high that you or someone you know has been consented to a pelvic exam—that's the extremely invasive one in which doctors examine the vulva, vagina, ovaries, uterus, rectum, and pelvis. Thinking back through my reproductive health-care history, I later realized this was not the first time. How many times had I allowed doctors to enter me with little questioning on my part or explanation on theirs because I wanted to be taken seriously, because I wanted to be OK? A cousin to being consented may be what writer Melissa Febos calls "empty consent," or a yes given "despite internal ambivalence, aversion, or revulsion." You're not forced, exactly, there's some agency. You aren't choosing either.

I removed my clothes, donned a gown, and awaited a pelvic exam. Ben held my hand. The nurse inserted her hand, to my discomfort. My eyes floated to the ceiling, dissociating from the intrusion. As I stared at the craggy ceiling panels, I hoped to not have a contraction while her fingers were inside me. She removed them. Nine centimeters! A winning number for admission. Relief swept over me. "What were you doing?" she asked, incredulous. "You should have been here hours ago."

Informed consent in healthcare means people are entitled to know the risks, benefits, and alternatives of a particular procedure or treatment. It is a right, both human and ethical, but it's also a law, according to Hermine Hayes-Klein, a lawyer who specializes in obstetric violence cases. "The law of informed consent and refusal is *the law*," she explained to me. "It's supposed to apply. When you go into a hospital, they hand you a patients' rights card. It's written on there. But culturally in obstetrics, it's ignored."

It's ignored for a litany of reasons. She tells me some. I infer others. Doctors are trained to act, not to ask. They rigidly follow hospital protocol. They fear being sued. They think they know better, or best. They train to manage emergent birth, not to support physiologic labor. They want to use what they know to do good by pregnant people and their kids. They are overworked, overwhelmed, and traumatized by their jobs. They're burned out.

But amid this onslaught we are losing our most fundamental human rights in perinatal care and childbirth, according to Hayes-Klein: the rights to autonomy, privacy, equal treatment, and nondiscrimination—or, as she puts it, "the right to make supported choices without other people's feelings about them curtailing those choices or making them more dangerous." The two prongs of informed consent—providing information and acquiring agreement—are violated frequently, Hayes-Klein says. "When the inform prong is violated, that can look like manipulation in the conversation, or misinformation. That happens often because the provider thinks they know what the person should do." As for consent, "you can't say yes if you don't also have the right to say no."

Pelvic exams top the list of procedures performed without the explicit consent of the person whose vagina is being entered. These exams have long been standard care. Providers consent pregnant people to them all the time. There are a few things to say about this reality. The first is that pelvic exams are an intimate and often uncomfortable experience, more so when you're pregnant. At least that was my experience. Providers walk into the room. Women are already gowned and pantsless. We hoist our feet into cold stirrups, legs akimbo, as we lie flattened on a table. We are then penetrated and examined, often without explanation. That's what being *consented to* means in practice. We go along with all of that because, well, the experts don't give us a choice, and we believe pelvic exams are necessary and safe. We wish to be helpful, not galling. And we pray to be healthy and not unwell.

"Hands speak more intimately than words," writes author André Aciman. He's discussing the deaf here, specifically his mother, but I immediately think about healthcare, about perinatal care specifically. Touch is intimate. It can excite, comfort, heal. It should also be welcome. It feels different to be touched when you have a being inside of you. When you are pregnant, you occupy a new body, one that is both familiar and strange. Entry to a person's body should occur by invitation only, never amid confusion, never by coercion.

A whopping fifty-two million pelvic exams were performed in the United States in 2015. However, experts say that they occur so frequently based on habit, not necessity. We've heard this song before. The pelvic exam's application in healthcare dates at least to ancient Rome. Doctors today believe they must touch a uterus before prescribing birth control. They want to measure dilation and effacement in the third trimester. It's your first time seeing a new provider—open your legs! There are countless reasons. We, in turn, assume we need these exams. We don't know we have a choice or that good evidence suggests that regular pelvic exams aren't necessary. Even during pregnancy. Especially during pregnancy. Rebecca Dekker of Evidence Based Birth said that research shows weekly cervical exams in pregnancy are "done more out of tradition and routine than anything else."

Often pelvic exams ramp up toward the end of pregnancy under the guise of providers guestimating how ready for labor you are. But this approach doesn't have a firm foothold in evidence. Of the two clinical trials that look at cervical checks in pregnancy, from 1984 and 1992, respectively, the first found that pelvic exams after thirty-seven weeks tripled the likelihood of a person's water breaking before labor began, while the second concluded pelvic exams provide "no harm or benefit." The harm point is subjective. But putting that aside for a moment, why are checks happening if they do no good? Measuring dilation and effacement provides no indication of when a baby will be born, and even though obstetricians admit this, they continue to check toward the end of pregnancy anyhow. Not only will measurements not predict a baby's arrival, but they might also encourage more intervention and invite coercive care. And yet I have never heard of a hospital that doesn't routinely conduct vaginal exams before admitting pregnant people. This isn't written policy, usually, but it is practiced faithfully.

There are midwives, doulas, and other birth attendants who believe the exam is unnecessary and even harmful. It can compromise the environment of the vagina, introducing bacteria into an otherwise perfectly healthy place. The more exams during a labor, the greater the chance of infection. Cervical checks often provide false information, creating expectations that dilation and birth will occur in a prescribed amount of time. Experienced midwives see people go from barely dilated to fully dilated and a baby being born very quickly (I was one of those people, twice) and also people holding steady at nine centimeters for many hours. Checking the cervix can put birthers "on a clock" in hospital parlance, leading to their being rushed unnecessarily or cornered into interventions they don't need or want. Checks can also invite doctors to perform a membrane sweep—loosening the amniotic sac from the uterus—which can start labor. This is often done without consent. Nonconsensual membrane stripping could explain why the 1984 study found a threefold greater chance of water breaking before labor begins.

Vaginal exams like cervical checks are ground zero for flagrant violations of consent. Penetrating a patient without their permission is battery. Doctors shouldn't do it—but they do, constantly. I've heard descriptions of patients who, while on the table, move their bodies away from the provider doing the exam. They close their legs, squirm, or appear visibly stricken or pained. They dissociate, like I did. I thought that was a tactic to withstand a pelvic exam, but upon reflection, I have realized it's an indication of nonconsent. In those moments, providers should stop, reset, and talk to the person on the table. That rarely happens.

My survey respondents and women I spoke to shared harrowing stories of being consented to traumatic exams. Lisa said, "The attending doctor gave me an internal examination in the middle of a contraction without warning or gaining my consent. It was the most painful part of my entire labor and deeply upsetting." I spoke to several women who recalled the pain and shame of doctors or residents conducting nonconsensual vaginal exams during contractions. May's doctor didn't ask. "She kept giving me vaginal exams even though I said they made me panic, and she didn't take my concerns seriously," she recalled.

Midwife and educator Stephanie Tillman reminds us that gynecology's history of misogyny, racism, and classism perfected "assault disguised as care." Contemporary pelvic care remains rife with these practices, "ranging from overt sexual assault to coercion disguised as guidance," she explains in a 2020 journal article. "If a patient does not believe they have consented to an examination or procedure, they are likely to rightfully identify with one of consent's antonyms, assault."

Evidence Based Birth, a leading birth educational resource, gives straightforward advice to avoid vaginal exams when you don't want them: remain dressed below the waist and say, "No, thank you." While I appreciate the tip, it also saddens me. We have to trick our doctors into not coercing us to perform vaginal exams we don't want by keeping our pants on when instructed to remove them. Instead of our refusal being reason enough, we have to say, "No, thank you," calling upon the skills we were taught as deferentially polite children. If we question or irritate our providers, we become a threat, and we could very likely face reprisal and punishment—coercion, assault, or withholding of desired care, as reports have shown. Meanwhile, the strongest weapon we wield to fight assault is the thin fabric of our pants.

MEDICAL PROFESSIONALS' WITHHOLDING OF INFORMED CONSENT and refusal is hardly limited to pelvic exams. Hayes-Klein gives another example: when a woman in labor sets a boundary that is ignored, or a provider steamrolls over her wishes using coercive tactics. A nurse pressures her into an IV, a Pitocin drip, an epidural, an episiotomy, abdominal surgery. Hayes-Klein points to doctors' statements like "Don't you care if your baby dies?" and "You want to be a good mother, right?" as typical of this category of abuse. Providers frequently manipulate birthing people and deprive them of their right to make decisions concerning their care by not offering them a choice.

"Every human has the right to make choices in their health care, to determine who touches them, like physically touches their body, what procedures and medications they have or don't have. Your rights are not suspended just because you're pregnant," says Cristen Pascucci, whose organization Birth Monopoly advocates for restoring human rights to childbirth. She believes those rights have been taken away. In pregnancy, choice is often revoked. Coercing people into birthing on their backs, not informing them of or offering evidence-based comfort measures, such as freely moving around and massage, denying food and water for hours or days, requiring constant fetal monitoring, and presenting any procedure, drug, or intervention as if it is the only option—these are all examples of forcing birthers to submit to providers' demands rather than following their own needs or preferences.

"We are now at the point where 'Do no harm' has no meaning anymore because we're assaulting people," said Tillman, the rare provider who will speak to this. "All of us have probably caused trauma to people, some more than others. How do we all do better?"

It's difficult to quantify how many people are deprived of choice, co-erced, manipulated, or assaulted during their childbirths. These aren't questions we routinely ask or an area that is thoroughly studied. Some 30 percent of my survey respondents said that during child-birth, they received procedures or care that they didn't want, con-sent to, or understand. From a list of adjectives used to describe their births, 40 percent chose "traumatic." Those who birthed in hospitals with obstetricians were more likely to receive care that they didn't consent to, and more likely to describe birth as "traumatic," than those who didn't.

Sadly, not everyone recognizes coercion, manipulation, or assault during birth even when they're experiencing it. I didn't. There's a lot going on! It's tough for people in active labor to hold a conversation, let alone weigh and make choices. Doulas I spoke to said their clients often believe abusive behavior is just part of the care. Cori Pleune, a Brooklyn-based doula, recalled an instance during the height of Covid in New York. Her client had planned a hospital birth but found herself with a crowning baby in the cab en route. Cori called to alert the hospital that they were coming and to describe what was happen-ing in the cab, so that staff would be prepared to receive her.

"I walk in with her, and I'm calmly holding the head, and like twenty-seven people rush us and just start pulling her legs apart," Cori recalled. After the baby was born, the woman complimented her care.

"But you wouldn't have wanted them to rush you and pull your legs apart like that, right?" Cori asked.

"Oh, right. Of course," the woman replied.

It's easy to misconstrue manipulation and abuse as good care during our own births. We walk into the delivery room believing that we have no expertise, that our all-knowing care providers will pilot us to shore. There is a cliché that demonstrates this phenomenon per-fectly: "In labor and delivery, you leave your rights at the door." In an-other version, it's "dignity" that's left there. Cristen Pascucci of Birth Monopoly hears this all the time from nurses, doctors, and even birth-ing people. "It's kind of like 'You come in here, we take over. You're just a passenger. We're in charge,'" she told me.

This mentality is present in what providers will "allow" birthers to do. I often hear this language when people describe the threat of induction—as in "My provider won't let me go past forty weeks." Phrasing the situation this way undermines the birther's expertise and authority. It puts the doctor firmly in charge before labor even begins. I've also often heard women use this framing when retelling the story of their C-sections: "My provider said he would only let me labor for a little bit longer before operating."

Tillman wants to teach every provider what proper consent and refusal look like. Consent to medical procedures surrounding labor and childbirth should mirror, if not exceed, the expectations and guidelines of any other intimate interaction in society, she writes. Crucially, she defines consent as a process that "equalizes the ability to respond either yes or no." For example, when a pregnant person questions an exam, a nudging response that doesn't invite dialogue might sound like "This is what we do for everyone" or "How else will we know if labor is progressing?"

Coercion sounds like this: "I hear you're declining, but I want to emphasize that . . . ," or "I know what's best," or, disgustingly, "I have to do this, or your baby will die." Forced examination or refusal to stop when asked—aka assault—sounds like this:

"You're doing great."

"Just another second."

"You will thank me later."

"I just need to check."

"Almost finished."

It's shocking how common such phrases are in perinatal care. I've heard instances of almost all of them being uttered, and I've heard some of them in my own healthcare.

Some providers take the informed consent crisis seriously and have begun to practice trauma-informed care, which acknowledges that every pregnant person has likely experienced some trauma in her life. At least one in four women has experienced rape or assault—far too many for doctors to ignore or discard their history. And yet they routinely do. I was in my thirties with two kids before a healthcare provider ever asked me whether I had experienced rape or sexual assault. She was a midwife. Tracey Vogel, an anesthesiologist also trained as a rape crisis counselor, told me that trauma-informed care, crucially, shifts power. "It takes us from 'I am your doctor, and this is what I'm going to be doing to you' to 'I want to know what you might need from me,'" she explained.

While more birth workers realize this shift is essential, Tillman laments that trauma-informed care is undermined when doctors believe there is an emergency, whether or not there actually is one. They tell her, "'Oh sure, I hear what you're saying about consent, and oh yeah, that's a good point; if someone closes their legs, maybe they've told me to stop.' But then you put it into these exceptional circumstances of emergencies, and everything goes out the window," she said in a podcast interview. Tillman, a midwife in Chicago, described an example of a birther experiencing cord prolapse, a very rare occurrence where the umbilical cord blocks the baby's passage. Providers believe that if the cord has prolapsed, they must insert their hand inside the vagina to move the cord and keep it there because that's what they were taught to do. "And so, if you're doing that cervical exam and you feel an umbilical cord, and, as you're doing that, the person gets a contraction and tells you to take your hand out, what do you do? And consistently providers say, 'You keep your hand in.' And that's not the right answer."

"Emergency" and "medical necessity" are murky categories. These terms are thrown around to use expertise to cudgel someone, even to force them. The idea that doctors know best and can act without pregnant peoples' consent is a baked-in societal bias. Cristen Pascucci sees it all the time when she's assisting obstetric-violence victims with finding legal aid.

"We're trying to hire a lawyer for somebody, and we say, 'This woman did not consent to this episiotomy. She said no,'" Pascucci told me. "And the lawyer says, 'Well, but wasn't it necessary?' And we go, 'That's literally beside the point, whether or not it was medically necessary. The point is that she didn't consent to it, so she never had the opportunity to decide whether or not that was necessary because nobody even talked to her about it. They just did it.' And the lawyer will say, 'I don't know. You know, episiotomies are necessary.' They literally can't even get past that cultural bias toward the consent piece, that you still have that consent right. It's really common." The belief that perceived emergency or necessity trumps consent can be insurmountable when a birthing person goes to court. Pascucci and Hayes-Klein both told me that jurors often display this bias.

Any patient can refuse any treatment, even one needed to maintain life, and pregnancy is not an exception, Pascucci wrote in an open letter to doctors. But she says that the common cultural assumption that pregnant people must submit to their doctors' decisions and whims threatens informed consent and stokes obstetric violence. It's difficult to say how many people who give birth in hospitals are fully exercising their rights to informed consent and refusal and retaining control of their own bodies. My guess is that almost no one is.

"THE PEOPLE WHO I'M SUPPOSED TO SHARE THIS STORY WITH TOLD me not to tell this story and tried to suppress this story. And those are the people who are responsible for keeping us safe when we have our babies." Barbie tells me this over the phone, as she is home with a six-month-old, her fourth child, who was born in the car. "I meant to make it," she says. I laugh at this because I can relate. But this isn't the story she wants to tell me now.*

Barbie, blonde and apple cheeked, had about six weeks of experience as a registered nurse when she began working labor and delivery at a Southern California hospital in December 2017. During one of her first days at work, she was paired with another nurse to observe a birth. They stood and chatted over the baby warmer as their more experienced colleagues assisted the doctor. Barbie appreciated how patient the provider was during the birth and told her colleague so. Her colleague agreed. Then her face changed. "Wait until you work with Dr. B," she said.

During her second week on the job, Barbie received a patient

---

* This section contains a graphic description of obstetric violence.

whose water had broken. Most hospitals want a contraction pattern to emerge quickly after that point, but it wasn't happening yet for this woman. Policies are "pretty restrictive," Barbie said: "We want you in, we want to monitor you and baby continuously." Her superiors ordered her to administer Pitocin immediately, even though the laboring woman hadn't asked for it. "I questioned it," Barbie told me, but the charge nurse persisted. Integral to rushing a labor is nestling an IV into a patient's arm. Since Barbie was new, she was "still being hazed. Trial by fire." If a new nurse like her couldn't land the intervention on the first or second try, a superior would finish the job—clean up after her, in a sense. "It's like, 'You're new, we want to throw you in there, sink or swim. Can you get these things done?' But also 'We need these interventions to happen. Make them happen.'"

"That's how nursing and medical education are set up. It's very violent. Patriarchy and white supremacy—they're in the care because they're layered into the education and training systems. I mean, all the way back to the beginning," she said. "At the cost of the patient."

Barbie dealt with this training style by often calling for help. "Because I don't like it ... using the patient as an experiment. I'd rather be looked at as a slow learner. Whatever to help the patient have a better experience." But that day, she landed the IV as she was asked, augmenting labor with Pitocin. The laboring woman accepted it but continued to refuse pain management, even though Pitocin-induced contractions can be brutal—far harder to tolerate than spontaneous ones. When the woman seemed ready to push, the nurses called Dr. B.

"It felt like a long time that he didn't show up," Barbie remembers. "My charge nurse told me to call him again." Dr. B finally arrived, in a rush, wearing a suit and tie. He didn't greet the patient. He removed his jacket, washed his hands, and put on gloves. "Let's have a baby," he said to the woman and four nurses in the room. One had prepared a tray of sterile instruments. The woman's partner was next to her.

"At this hospital it was common practice to either coerce or just make it not seem like a choice, to encourage patients to give birth on their backs," Barbie said. This reduces the pelvic opening significantly and makes birth harder and tearing easier. When a woman births on her back, neither she nor her partner can see what the providers are doing below.

Like most hospitals, Barbie's encouraged coached or "closed glottis" pushing: count to ten, hold your breath, push. There's good evidence (which I'll present in Chapter 11) that it shouldn't be as common as it is. It reduces oxygen supply to mom and baby. Withholding oxygen from someone working very hard is a terrible idea. People can pass out. Depriving oxygen can cause fetal heart rate monitors to pick up distressing tones, spurring unnecessary intervention. Despite the kind of pushing that can harm all involved, mom and baby were chugging along.

"There was nothing emergent," Barbie stressed.

She described what happened next: Dr. B inserted his left hand into the vaginal opening and started pressing down. The perineum was fully stretched around the baby's head. The baby's head was crowning, and the baby was about to come out. Barbie thought that after a few more pushes they would all meet the baby. Instead, Dr. B "takes his left hand and carves the perineal tissue. He grasps it with his left hand and pinches it. The perineal skin is very taut, almost like a thick piece of paper. He takes his right hand, and he pinches and just rips the perineum down toward her anus." I gasp on the phone. I've read that quote a lot, but I still shudder every time.

The woman screamed.

When I ask Barbie what manual tearing is, she says, "It's nothing. It's not a procedure. It's not an intervention. We don't collect data on it. It's ripping the perineum. It's medical battery." When she witnessed Dr. B assaulting her patient, she tells me, she knew exactly what she had seen.

"The image of her flesh hanging like that when he let go, before the baby was born, is very much imprinted." One of her colleagues stepped back, stiff against a wall and staring. Her supervisor "looked more angry than disgusted."

But Barbie couldn't focus on the assault. She jumped into response mode—caring for the baby. Her nursing pedagogy hadn't included advice on what to do when witnessing a doctor assaulting a patient. And it wasn't over.

The woman and her partner had been reveling in the warm baby on their chest for a few minutes when Dr. B began pulling on the umbilical cord, trying to force out the placenta. Severe fundal pressure (pressing the top of the uterus) is sometimes needed in emergencies when the placenta must come out fast, but that's not what this was, Barbie said. Most placentas exit on their own. The woman and her partner were bonding with the baby, who was latching, so they weren't paying attention to what was going on at the bottom of the table.

"Then he sticks his middle finger into her anus and kind of wiggles it. She jumps. He says, 'Oh, I'm just checking to see if baby tore you all the way through.'" Barbie said that Dr. B was used to epiduralized patients who wouldn't have been able to feel what he was doing.

"At that moment, I have my reality check. This guy just seriously assaulted this patient right in front of all of us. And the patient and her partner don't even know."

Barbie left the room and overheard Dr. B record what occurred as a second-decree laceration, meaning, it happened naturally. "That's fraud in the electronic health record," she said. Later, she decided to file her own report. She wrote that Dr. B had manually torn an episiotomy in the perineum with his hands and without consent. A supervisor fought with her about it and convinced her to simply call it a "laceration." "It was institutional gaslighting," Barbie said.

"She also asked me to remove that there was no consent, just write what he had done. So, the patient record is a laceration with a comment that he manually tore her. I wasn't able to get any other information in there like I wanted, that it was done without consent and that there was no communicated clinical distress." Meaning it was done needlessly.

Once the report was filed, Barbie returned to the bedside. The new mother had sensed that something was wrong. She asked whether she tore. "I told her, 'You didn't tear. Dr. B decided to tear you. If you have any questions about why he did that, you should ask him.'" Barbie added that she should see a pelvic floor physical therapist, later, to make sure she was healing properly. The mom thanked Barbie, who never saw her again.

It was a practiced assault, Barbie said, concealed by two lies. The first lie was that the baby tore her when the doctor did. The second was that what had occurred was a natural laceration, as the doctor stated in his report. Barbie believes the battery was a workaround—a way to do an episiotomy without doing an episiotomy. Hospitals record episiotomies because they are surgeries. When their surgical birth rates are too high, insurers can spike their premiums or threaten their coverage. They don't want to pay for anything they don't have to pay for.

The reported episiotomy rate at Barbie's hospital has dropped in recent years. It is around 2.5 percent, down from 4 percent in 2019 and 7 percent in 2015. One reason for the plunge is that data-savvy groups like patient collaboratives, healthcare advocates, and consumer organizations are increasingly scrutinizing hospital birth practices, especially costly surgeries. Barbie said her hospital had been pushing to lower episiotomy and cesarean rates for fear of censure by watchdogs like these. Around the time she began her job, she remembers discovering that Dr. B had an incredibly high episiotomy rate. That was in 2016, and his rate was "probably in the seventieth percentile"—but then "it dropped very, very low," she said. "Like well below 10 percent. And then his second- and third-degree laceration rate flipped. It went really high. Almost 90 percent. Whether they were tearing by accident, or he was doing it to as many people as possible, I don't know," she said. I reached out to the hospital, but they wouldn't confirm Dr. B's episiotomy rates.

There are evidence-based labor practices to help doctors lower their episiotomy rates. The proper procedure is first to explain, to get consent. Asking permission to cut lowers rates because people don't want the procedure. "Rarely is an emergency such an emergency that we don't have time to explain that there is an emergency," Barbie said. But from where Barbie was sitting, the baby was coming, nearly there. There was no emergency. An episiotomy was pointless, gratuitous. Battery, assault.

Barbie learned from her coworkers later that what Dr. B had done occurred frequently enough to have a nickname: the B Maneuver.

Some nurses said, "Well, women tear anyway, so it doesn't matter." Others had tried reporting him but concluded that their efforts never produced results, that he was untouchable. Still others refused to talk about it. Barbie would bring it up; they would shift uncomfortably and change the subject. One nurse saw Dr. B tear people so routinely that she believed the act to be a part of normal care. I had wondered that myself, so I asked midwives and OBGYNs about it. Is there such a procedure as manual tearing? Resounding nos.

Weeks after she had first witnessed the assault, Barbie tried filing another report. An administrator read it and asked to see her. She said that Dr. B was within his rights, that he was just trying to save the patient another twenty minutes of pushing because it was her first baby. "I remember these little alarm bells," Barbie said. "This is not the right response." Barbie was disenchanted and growing scared. She also had no guarantee that the B Maneuver wouldn't happen again.

Barbie adapted her behavior when she worked with Dr. B. She waited until the last possible minute to call him to a birth. She used her own body to block his path to women. "I would physically not allow him access to the perineum by either using my own hand or a warm compress or positioning myself in his way, so that he would have to ask me to move." She didn't want to give him any space to assault a patient. It was incredibly stressful. She also spent time explaining consent to birthers when he was in the room. Dr. B would rush birthers, telling them he "had to get going." Barbie would say the opposite: "You have plenty of time. There are other doctors." If she was attending someone who had given birth before, Barbie would ask about their previous experience. She would say, "'Hey, did you tear before?' And I would very clearly state when Dr. B came in the room, 'They didn't tear last time. Isn't that great?'"

Despite Barbie's reports and meetings with leadership, Dr. B wasn't reprimanded. He still practices. She doesn't work at the hospital anymore—the environment was too stressful, its location too far from home.

WHAT BARBIE SHARED MADE ME REALIZE, FOR THE FIRST TIME, the coercion and abuse that had been present in my own births. As a laboring person, it's hard to know whether the resident or nurse trainee is capable and caring or is following orders to do something to your body, to rush your labor because of hospital quotas and conventions, with or without your consent. I gave birth on my back when I tore. But after listening to Barbie, I realize that I didn't remember choosing to be in that position. Who chose for me?

I was admitted to the hospital after the cervical check that I was consented to. I paced around one of the precious, income-generating labor and delivery rooms. That is, until the rookie nurse arrived. Her supervisor instructed her to insert the IV into me. I didn't want one. She bothered me until I agreed. She couldn't find the vein. But that didn't stop her from trying. And trying and trying, until my arm was black and blue. Not long after, the needle bulging from my arm bothered me more than the cresting contractions. I nudged until she removed it. She was reprimanded by her charge nurse. Days later, when I went home with my baby, the needle-pricked place on my arm swelled like the inside of a plum.

After the needle was inserted and then removed, my doctor asked if he could break my water. I had been at the hospital for a couple of hours, on a federal holiday, and it was getting dark outside. I said, "No, thank you," slightly irritated that he forgot or hadn't read my birth plan, but began doubting myself as soon as he left. Would the baby come right away if he did that? I was just a few hours from giving birth on the same day that my first child was born, and I felt strongly that they shouldn't share a birthday. I was also getting tired, anxious, and eager to meet my baby. I consulted my doula, Sarah. Maybe I wanted to take him up on his offer? I didn't have that much time to think about it. Not long after he had first visited, the doctor came back again. "We can break your water," he said a second time. I knew at my core that I didn't want this, but his pestering was getting in my head. It made me doubt myself.

When we're laboring, do we know and trust that we have a right to have preferences? To have opinions? To say no? He was just asking.

There was no harm in the suggestion. But it felt coercive. I had stated to him in person and on paper that I specifically didn't want my membranes ruptured. I had declined cervical checks during my entire pregnancy. I liked my doctor, but when he offered to break my water a second time, it made me feel as if the person who was supposed to help me birth my child wasn't listening to me and didn't respect my wishes. I felt rushed, one of many pregnant ladies pumped down the conveyer belt, taking up a valuable, cash-generating room. In the end, I didn't do it. But there is a world in which I might have.

THE GOAL IS HUMAN RIGHTS IN CHILDBIRTH—EVERY BIRTHING person at the center of their care and experience. Advocates like Pascucci believe this is achievable. All birthing people should decide where, how, and with whom to birth. Midwifery care, particularly the kind that exists outside hospitals, is bound by an ethos that centers birthers in their own care. It's a model obstetricians should follow. Doula support in any birth setting is integral to the solution. They are uniquely positioned to advocate for birthers and don't answer to hospitals.

I asked Pascucci what it would look like if we achieved this—everyone centered in their care. She paused.

"I think it looks like a reduction in procedure rate, a dramatic lowering of trauma-related diagnoses and symptoms," she said. "It looks like a lowering of the maternal mortality rate because these things all feed into one another. You can't separate out disrespect and abuse from poor health outcomes. They're all part of the same package when you're not listening to people. That's why you're not catching hemorrhages. If you're forcing risky care on people, there is a reason they would decline that care. Because they have their own best interest in mind."

What Pascucci describes is a complete shift in who has the power in childbirth.

The moment my baby was out, I wanted to be at home, but it would be almost forty-eight hours before I walked through my front door. I remember thinking that if I ever did this again, it wouldn't be here, at the hospital. I would do it at home. And when I became pregnant with my third kid, these seemingly small moments of nonconsent replayed in my mind—the obligatory pelvic exam, the needle in my arm, the bruise like rotten fruit, the lithotomy position someone put me in both times. Sure, both births were beautiful, vaginal, *natural*—tick, tick, tick on the boxes of imaginary birth "success." But these were the moments I couldn't shake, that wedged themselves in and made me angry, ill. I had gaslit myself not to have a home birth. What if I need the NICU? I thought the first time. A big reason I had rejected having a home birth with my second child was my fear of the upstairs neighbors hearing us. The sweet couple whose children had moved away. I didn't want my moans drifting up to disturb them. Even though Ben and our amazing doulas were convinced I should do it, I said no. I didn't want to make a mess, to rely on someone else to clean it up.

During my third pregnancy I didn't care about any of this anymore. I didn't want my body to be forced to birth in a doctor-designed position. I didn't want to remain trapped in a hospital, after my baby was born, bothering and fighting just to leave when they needed to keep me for insurance purposes. I wanted it my way, on my turf, next time.

CHAPTER 8
MUMMY TUMMY

I AM LYING ON MY BACK ATOP A PADDED TABLE. ON THE INTERIOR treatment room wall hangs a pair of abstract paintings featuring thick bands of green, purple, and muted gold. They are Mardi Gras colors and appear vaguely vaginal. My gaze catches a Costco-sized bottle of lubricant on a small cart. Music that sounds like chanting blends with the air conditioning fan. Here I am again, postpartum, for the third time. The birth of my third child had been transformative, wholly new. It's a story I'll return to later. Here, I'm sweaty with hormone turnover, prostrate without pants.

By now, I know to be evaluated by a pelvic floor physical therapist. I did not know this after my first birth. I went far too long without knowing. Perhaps this is because when the pelvic floor functions as it should, we don't think about it at all. It is through discord, through dysfunction, that the pelvic floor becomes known to us.

Before pregnancy, all I knew about the pelvic floor was that I could lift it during intercourse or a yoga class. The boutique fitness studios I favored for more than a decade evangelized about the "Kegel," so I did them in spades. But my first brush with the exercise had been as a teenager in the Kroger checkout line. There, magazine covers offered enticing promises like "How to Enslave a Man and Make Him Yours for Life" and "Make Him Beg for It." The accompanying articles described Kegels as the feeling of stopping your pee flow. They claimed that practicing lift would make you better at sex. Through the lens of 1990s women's magazines, Kegels belonged to a self-betterment routine, like juicing or Botox. They improved a shoddy, ready-to-fail body part, increasing attractiveness. They were vagina-tightening work to please men.

Michele is a pelvic health specialist from Northern Ireland who practices in Brooklyn. Her approach to Kegels is radically different than early-aughts *Cosmopolitan*. As I'm lying on the table, she tells me that the pelvic floor moves all the time—to bend, hold things aloft, run, jump. When it's working as designed, it's lightly contracting nonstop. Postpartum women are a large subset of Michele's patients. She examines externally and internally to gauge the pelvic floor's strength and ability to move, hence my pantslessness. We discuss what checking my pelvic tone will entail. Are the muscles firing as they should? Are they weak? Is there any leakage or pain?

With my consent, Michele inserts gloved fingers. She tells me to visualize the four corners of my pelvis elevating. I imagine the points of a scarf and the word *flutter*. Then, an image from childhood—the animated bluebirds carrying the tablecloth in *Snow White*. I don't feel four corners or any connection to my musculature. My pelvic floor must be there, but it's not responding to the imagery. Maybe it flickers, but it doesn't lift.

"Now, picture an elevator," she says, "rising to higher and higher floors. Let's go to eight."

I conjure the metal box in a lobby with its buttons and lights. Next comes the destabilizing feeling of the box moving, gaining momentum, shooting up to the rafters. I understand that the lift she's asking for must build on itself now. Higher and higher. I close my eyes and attempt to move my internal pelvic elevator upward. It gets stuck. I can't hold onto the contraction. The bluebird blanket wafts to the ground.

BACK IN MY FIRST WEEKS AS A NEW MOTHER, I CLUNG TO THE IDEA that the six-week postpartum visit would right what was newly wrong. I had been ushered out of the hospital forty-eight hours after birth and into a radically different life. I found myself in physical dislocation and identity disarray. During the so-called fourth trimester, I was exhausted, depleted, bleeding, in pain, and desperate for someone to help my beleaguered body and soul. I was holding two desires: I wanted to hear that I was fine, and I wanted someone to *see*—to witness and validate my upheaval.

When we're baby receptacles, we're coddled and cared for. Specialists spend months surveilling our pregnant forms. Naturally, we assume some version of this treatment will continue postpartum. Especially those of us who give birth in hospitals laden with people attending patients. We don't realize that once the baby is out, so are we. Overnight, we go from being meticulously observed to totally ignored. Obstetrician Alison Stuebe gave me a potent analogy: "America treats new moms like candy wrappers: Once the candy is out of the wrapper, the wrapper is thrown away."

Postpartum people experience a long list of typical symptoms in the first week after childbirth: lochia (heavy bleeding), abdominal cramping, constipation, hemorrhoids, night sweats, chills, elimination struggles, engorged breasts and breast pain, back pain, headaches, body aches, perineal pain, incision pain, difficulty walking (from an episiotomy or tearing), depression, anxiety, and exhaustion. More serious and rarer postpartum complications include hemorrhage, incontinence, symphysis pubis dysfunction (extreme pain in the pelvic girdle), and pelvic organ prolapse (when organs like the uterus or bladder slip down into the vagina).

For postpartum women, most if not all of this is unexpected. "There's this fantasy. Your body is going to come back together. Your organs are going to be in place. It's an illusion," pelvic floor physical therapist Isa Herrera told me. "I find almost no education about what will happen in the postpartum period. I tell pregnant women what is going to happen and what to do about it instead of saying, basically, 'You're screwed.'"

In Listening to Mothers, half of women reported pain in the weeks after birth. In fact, the most common health problem within the first two months postpartum was incision pain among those who birthed surgically—58 percent experienced it; 19 percent called it "a major problem." Some 41 percent of women who birthed vaginally reported pain in the perineum, "a finding strongly related to whether or not a mother experienced an episiotomy," according to study authors. Close to 80 percent of new moms agreed that postpartum pain interfered with their daily activities. A third reported struggles using the bathroom. The pandemic has winnowed the already short postpartum hospital stay even further: in the summer of 2020, 73 percent of hospitals sent moms and babies home less than forty-eight hours after birth, according to the Centers for Disease Control and Prevention.

Providers encourage us to wait for that six-week visit to share health concerns (as they dismiss questions with an eye roll and the pejorative "Don't read the internet"). The specialist new moms see immediately is the pediatrician who cares for their baby but not for them. A quarter of mothers return to work two weeks after delivery. Some 40 percent of my survey respondents agreed that doctors, nurses, and specialists didn't give them the postpartum care they needed. Our bodies and well-being are not just deprioritized, they're irrelevant.

The six-week checkup is highly anticipated but laughably insufficient. During the checkup, the provider who delivered the baby examines a woman's vagina and breasts and, if applicable, her C-section incision. They palpate the uterus, which should have returned to its original size. They offer birth control and greenlight sex and exercise. That's it. In my survey, postpartum moms reported receiving general information during the six-week checkup, but as one respondent put it, "They don't talk to you." Thus, among postpartum women, the six-week checkup is as mythologized as it is useless. There's only one postpartum visit because that's what insurers will cover. Providers aren't incentivized to give care they aren't paid for. They're overworked as it is.

Why the checkup occurs when it does—at the six-week mark—appears to be more cultural than medical. Stuebe, the obstetrician who first pointed me toward this idea, reminded me that in the Bible, Jesus was brought to the Temple forty days after his birth. Many non-Western cultures historically and today adhere to a thirty- to forty-day lying-in period for babies and moms. In China, it's called confinement. In Mexico, it's called curanteña. Family members attend to new mothers with special foods and restorative body work. They handle chores and childcare so the mother can rest. American moms could benefit from these customs, but instead they trudge to a doctor's office six weeks later. Even to experts, the delay is ridiculous. Stuebe said, "Waiting forty days to check in doesn't make sense."

Moms and babies have needs after birth that emerge over time. Researcher Kristin Tully and her colleagues at the University of North Carolina's 4th Trimester Project spent two years following postpartum women and health professionals who care for them. They learned that women were too ashamed to talk about symptoms that weren't broached with them first. They also didn't know what treatments could help. "Women didn't know the range of what's normal, when to seek guidance, and whom to ask," Tully told me.

This doesn't surprise me. The books I read when I was pregnant hardly mentioned the postpartum period. Some briefly explained the six-week checkup, but that was it. Nurses warned about baseball-sized blood clots that could mean hemorrhage and implored me to call if I saw one. They didn't mention that it was normal to bleed for weeks. Even if I had known to anticipate it all, expectations aren't the same as experience. Knowing you might suffer isn't suffering.

"Postpartum care isn't ingrained in US medicine," said the OBGYN at my postpartum visit, who caught my second child with one hand. "It never was. The medical system was never geared to help the well, only the sick. Look at you. Someone like you. You look well; you're doing great. You could easily slip through the cracks."

My first six-week exam was brief. Shorter than the coffee line I waited in beforehand. It didn't validate my struggles. I don't even remember whether my midwife looked to see if my tear had healed. She did permit me to have sex and exercise again. At this point, feeding and nurturing a baby was consuming not only my being but my body. I was ready to take it back. I wanted to move but, if I'm honest, mostly in service of improving my appearance. A protruding stomach was fine with a baby inside, but now that she was out, it was odious to me. I wanted to tighten my midsection. Reclaim the contents of my closet. Find the quickest path to losing ten pounds.

I told the instructor at barre class that I had recently given birth and didn't feel connected to my core. She said that I was in the right place: crunches would sculpt my soft stomach—do lots! I believed I needed to be tighter, firmer, and smaller—snapping back to the body I'd inhabited before housing a human, into a body like those I saw selling things—board flat, unblemished. Media stomachs never sagged or looked dappled, like ripples in a lake. I jogged along the Brooklyn docks and took barre classes, costly bastardizations of my girlhood pastime, ballet. Instead of feeling strong and content afterword, I felt shaky and unmoored in my center, and my back routinely ached.

Ben and I flew across country with our baby just before her first birthday. We schlepped bags. Rode trams. Stuffed into cars. I wore her in a carrier all day, straps contorting my torso. Twenty-four hours after a bad airport Shake Shack burger, my stomach rejected its contents and refused further admission. For a full day, I only vomited and slept. The day after that, I herniated a disc in my back. It seemed to seep hot fluid down my entire left side. Walking hurt, sitting hurt. I couldn't find a position to put my body in that didn't light it up with pain. I limped around San Francisco, alternating between ice and heat, eating ibuprofen, and numbing with Biofreeze and Tiger Balm. The only relief came with being unconscious when I was finally able to sleep. My body had never felt so wrong. Later, an osteopath told me that stomach illness can compromise musculature. Forces shooting everywhere. No wonder.

I called my physician, the one I'd vowed to replace, desperate for something stronger than hotel packets of ibuprofen. He said no by way of reminding me that ibuprofen was potent enough, and hadn't I had a natural childbirth? Couldn't I withstand this until I was back home and able to come to the office?

Two back surgeons wanted to operate on me. One of them offered a slot later that week. Why wait? he asked. You're a mess.

I didn't realize how long I had endured the pain until recently when I turned to a journal I kept from that time. Each entry documented what my first baby did: eat steamed carrots, babble sounds, move limbs. I'm a ghost in the pages. It's my lens, but I'm barely there. However, I appear briefly in an entry from her first birthday: "I've been in pain practically the whole first year of her life," I wrote. I had forgotten how much and how often I'd hurt before the disc blew.

I felt like I needed to address the crippling pain before figuring out its cause, and I avoided back surgery by getting an epidural steroid injection. It was Michele's therapy combined with rehabilitative Pilates that ultimately revealed the cause of my injury. While I'd been slathering on all manner of creams and balms to prevent stretch marks and doing a million crunches to tighten my abs, I hadn't noticed that the place where my abdominal muscles had separated during pregnancy had left, essentially, a gaping hole that didn't close after birth. I was working on the outside while the inside couldn't hold.

THE CORE IS A MAGNET FOR TOXIC DIET CULTURE. IT'S DISCUSSED and treated in isolation—"Apply the stretch mark cream!" and "Do crunches!" But it is integral to effective bodily function because of its relationship to other parts. It holds you up.

Picture a canister. The pelvic floor is the bottom, the diaphragm is the top, and the transverse abdominus, or the muscles of the abdominal corset, form the front and back. These groups of muscles collaborate with each breath we take. This is why a change or something malfunctioning in the abdomen, such as the abdominal separation common to pregnancy and childbirth, can compromise our movement, breathing, elimination, and sexual pleasure.

I assumed that the muscles, ligaments, tissues, and bones that shifted and lengthened to house my baby would all snap back to their previous sizes and places. I didn't realize that this doesn't always happen, that the body can take a different path or outright refuse to be what it was before. All pregnancies require some degree of abdominal separation, but sometimes the muscles cleave too much and the gaping persists past pregnancy. I didn't know about this possibility until it happened to me. I had heard about abdominal strain from a Pilates teacher friend who was pregnant when I was, but I didn't take the concern seriously. I believed that because I was young and healthy, I was unlikely to experience anything that sounded so weird. I resumed my online stroller research. Tellingly, it didn't register that "mom pooch," "baby belly," and "mummy tummy," phrases I was absolutely hearing (and fearing) from pregnancy books, were all related to what the Pilates teacher was trying to tell me. I figured that these terms just referred to a failure to lose weight. I didn't know they were related to a functional disorder.

Diastasis recti (DR) is the clinical name for abdominal separation caused by the overstretching of the linea alba, a fibrous structure that runs perpendicularly between the rectus abdominis muscles, holding them together. Linea alba is Latin for "white line." This channel runs the length of the torso, starting from the base of the sternum, bisecting the navel, and extending down to the pubis symphysis, at the bottom of the pelvis. It's stretchy, allowing the body to fold, twist, and shelter a fetus. The forces of stretching and pressure during pregnancy, however, can extend the linea alba so much that it doesn't resume its prior position. In her book about the condition, biomechanist Katy Bowman gives the analogy of a shirt seam. The linea alba connects to muscles the way seams hold together clothing. Seams are strong, but also weak, in that they are prone to tearing. The linea alba, too, is strong, but being a connector makes it more likely to rip or gape apart.

Bowman points out that the linea alba isn't an independent body holding things together so much as it is formed by the interconnecting muscles. Pelvis, ribcage, rectus abdominis, hips, and waist all pull on it. "Almost all motions of the body, even those 'outside' the core, *directly tug* on the core," she explains. Overstretching the linea alba from pregnancy, combined with movement of any kind elsewhere in the body, can cause the midsection to bulge or dome.

This round middle phenomenon is anathema in the consumer diet and fitness gulag. If DR is merely a cosmetic flaw, then diet culture and products can fix and perfect it—smoothing wrinkles, flattening protrusion, melting away unseemly fat. That's how media coverage of DR goes. By representing the postpartum belly as a problem of appearance, rather than function, the diet and exercise industries portray DR as something they can fix.

The media focus on appearance is loud and clear in headlines that plead, for example, "It's Never Too Late to Fix a Mom Pooch," or "Here's How to Lose That Mummy Tummy." "You can easily expect to see 2 inches off your waist in three weeks of time. That's not an unrealistic expectation," explained Leah Keller, founder of a workout promising to correct the problem that was featured in an NPR story titled "Flattening the Mummy Tummy with One Exercise 10 Minutes a Day." Keller taught women and the reporter Michaeleen Doucleff her exercises, then whipped out her measuring tape to chart "belly circumference" and (hopefully) shrinkage. Women and physical therapists criticized the piece, claiming it missed the point and fueled the problem of treating postpartum bodies like projects. A follow-up aired some of these grievances. Two members of the board of the American Physical Therapists Association wrote that "postpartum rehabilitation is a multi-muscle, integrative process, not as simple as the 'One muscle/one exercise' approach proposed in the story." The story "reinforced damaging cultural standards about women's bodies," explained a dietician in Austin, Texas, who thought it skirted an opportunity to "change the conversation about women's bodies to make it about function rather than aesthetics."

DR is both common and hidden. Some 60 percent of women have a separation six weeks after birth, and 30 percent still do a year later. They aren't screened for it at the postpartum visit, and most women have never heard of the condition.

Take Jenna, a mom of two in Atlanta. After her son was born, she was frustrated by the "mom pooch" in her midsection that lingered after she had returned to her prepregnancy weight. She lifted her shirt at her OB's office to reveal her stomach. "I said, 'What's this? Look at this.' She laughed at me," Jenna said. "I see why this bothers you," her OB said. "This is purely aesthetic. This is something you might have to deal with but if you do surgery, you'll have a big scar. Would you rather have a flat stomach and a huge scar?" This was only one of the doctors who brushed her off, accusing her of vanity.

"I found it appalling that I had to go on such a journey to get answers—talking to friends, to my OB, to a physical therapist and four plastic surgeons, who all told me DR couldn't be cured with physical therapy," Jenna told me. "The information is not readily available. It wasn't until well after my son's first birthday that I had some answers."

Because we're taught to loathe "jelly belly" and hang our worth on the pursuit of washboard abs, we treat DR as a surface-level problem and miss the underlying cause entirely. My stomach didn't sag; thus, DR wasn't visible to me at all. The outward appearance of my midsection hooked my attention, distracting me from what was inside. I only discovered the DR after suffering tremendous pain in a different part of my body. No one checked me for a separation at six weeks postpartum, which is what experts recommend. The back specialists I saw didn't consider my front.

The real danger of DR isn't the pouch in your middle, it's the problems it can cause elsewhere. I've continued to see Michele, the Brooklyn physical therapist and osteopath, since my disc herniation years ago. Through physical therapy, along with the epidural steroid injection, I avoided surgery. I started to talk to Michele about postpartum injury and recovery as I was lying on her table staring at the ceiling all those hours, being treated for both abdominal separation and pelvic floor dysfunction. Together we assembled the puzzle pieces: the back injury was old, but it was also connected to the instability in the front and the related pelvic floor weakness.

DR is commonly measured in finger widths. To check for it, I exhale deeply, then lift my neck and shoulders off of the table, while she

palpates my middle with her fingers. She can slide two fingers between my abdominal muscles, and there is a little extra room, but not
quite enough for a third. Some people also look at depth—how far
the fingers go down. Ultrasound machines get the most accurate measurements for DR. Michele has used that on me, too, applying the ge-
latinous substance I associate with seeing my babies for the first time
and then running the wand across my navel as she cues me to contract
my core. We can see on the screen which muscles are firing, which
aren't, and how the bands of muscle glide against one another. Sometimes it takes a few repetitions for the stagnant portions to flicker.

Michele doesn't think separation itself is clinically relevant unless
it's causing a functional hurdle. "One of my primary concerns is to get
the proper muscles firing," she tells me. "Are you feeling the two sides
of the transverse abdominus glide together? For the majority of postpartum women, it's not happening, or it's asymmetrical." Separations
spanning more than two finger widths, she says, often result in dysfunction, and that's what she seeks to treat. Many patients come to her
because they're leaking urine when they cough or sneeze, and when
she checks for a separation, she's often the first person to find one.

Pelvic health assessment to check for, diagnose, and treat DR and
other postpartum conditions should be routine. However, because
our healthcare system discards the candy wrapper once the treat is
free, this is not the case. We postpartum moms can't diagnose ourselves, so instead of securing help so we can live and breathe normally, we simply go on the best we can. Postpartum care is treated
as a privilege rather than a necessity. Where healthcare fails, diet
and fitness culture creep in. They fragment our bodies into fixable
parts—abs! pelvic floor!—and prescribe isolated exercises and diets, many invented by men and branded by corporations, to slim and
"improve" us.

Sara Reardon, a pelvic specialist who treats patients in New Orleans, said that about two-thirds of women have DR during pregnancy,
and a third do after, but health professionals miss their cases. "These
women aren't getting sent to therapy," she told me. "It's like, 'Oh this
is normal.' But they could be doing crunches or crazy exercises or

getting out of bed with shitty posture. And nobody's telling them, 'Hey, that would be making DR worse or that could be preventing it from getting better.' It's such a common condition, but women aren't getting referred to therapy to help with that."

Pelvic dysfunction accompanies DR more often than not. A survey of urogynecology patients found that 66 percent of women diagnosed with DR also had a form of pelvic floor dysfunction, such as incontinence or organ prolapse. But we aren't taught about this part of the body when it's healthy. We suffer first. Sometimes we come to realize this part hasn't functioned properly all along.

The pelvic floor isn't just mysterious to its owners. It's commonly overlooked by specialists in traditional fields of medicine. "Gynecologists, urologists and colorectal surgeons concentrate on their areas of interest and tend to ignore the pelvic floor common to them all," explains Kari Bø, a pelvic floor expert at the Norwegian School of Sports Science. Doctors in those fields see only their own specialty's area of the pelvis (or hole in the pelvis), whereas Bø encourages care for the "whole pelvis."

The pelvic floor isn't a single muscle. It's actually a three-layered sling composed of nerves, connective tissue called fascia, ligaments, tendons, and blood vessels. Pelvic floor muscles connect to pelvic bones in three places: the pubic joint in the front, the coccyx, or tailbone, in the back, and a pair of sitz bones (or ischial tuberosity) on the left and right. It's a hammock, a harness, a trampoline. The pelvic floor is springy, pliable, and taut, strong enough to support your organs, posture, and waist, and supple enough to fill with breath and to move as you do.

Pelvic floor disharmony can take many forms: Pain when you walk. The menstrual cup or tampon won't stay put. Intercourse hurts. Orgasm is weak or elusive. You squirt pee when you cough or laugh. A weak anal sphincter results in leakage. You have a feeling of uncomfortable fullness as organs drop into the vagina (where they are definitely not meant to go). About a quarter of women have pelvic floor disorders, which researchers describe as "a cluster of health problems that causes physical discomfort and limits activity," according to the National Institutes of Health. The three main disorders are urinary incontinence, fecal incontinence, and pelvic organ prolapse. Many of these symptoms and conditions also occur in DR patients, as the conditions are interlinked.

The more babies women have, the greater the odds of pelvic ailment. A study published in the *Journal of the American Medical Association* found pelvic floor disorder in 18 percent of US women with one child, 25 percent of women with two, and 32 percent of women with three or more. The study only captured women with moderate or severe disorder, meaning these numbers are high, and yet they likely undercount. Pelvic floor physical therapists say many women don't know they have pelvic floor symptoms and disorders.

The incidence of pelvic floor disorders begins after childbirth and escalates as women age. Researchers at the National Institutes of Health identified at least one pelvic floor disorder in 10 percent of women aged twenty to thirty-nine, in 27 percent of those aged forty to fifty-nine, in 37 percent of the sixty to seventy-nine demographic, and in 50 percent of women older than eighty. This 2008 report was the first to document the extent of pelvic floor disorders in US women.

Globally, most women have babies, and it seems that a high percentage of them are still suffering postpartum injuries long after their births. Urine leakage starts with the pelvic floor. One doctor told me that families commonly give up on caring for their aging loved ones when they lose bladder control. Kids don't want to change their parents' diapers. Urinary incontinence is a leading cause of nursing home admissions for women. This means that whether or not you can live your final days independently may come down to what's unresolved from giving birth, in a part of your body you don't really understand or might not even know is there.

The healthcare system isn't just failing postpartum women. It's failing women of all ages for their entire lives.

As with DR, the pelvic floor's condition isn't routinely assessed during the six-week postpartum visit. Say the words *pelvic floor* to an obstetrician, and usually the best answer they can muster is "Do

Kegels!" But "Do Kegels" isn't helpful, said Christa, a mom of two in Atlanta who took my survey. Instead, she wished that her doctor, or someone, anyone, had explained the pelvic floor and how to maintain it. When a Portland mom, Nicola, told her doctor that sex was excruciatingly painful and her body felt broken, the only prescription offered was Kegels "multiple times a day," she told *New York* magazine's *The Cut*. Kegels are what mothers "hear we 'should' be doing quickly after birth," said Carmen in Berkeley, but she believes her postpartum time was better spent resting. Karin's doctor told her that Kegels would solve her incontinence problem and showed her how to download an instructional app.

Kegels are "a flimsy replacement for comprehensive care for women," the article continues. "The problem is that Kegels don't work all that well, and many doctors aren't recommending any other treatments." Like abdominal crunches, Kegels can be part of a holistic approach to healing and strengthening the body after childbirth. But also like crunches, they won't work in isolation.

Gynecologist Arnold Kegel gets the credit for inventing modern pelvic floor exercise and therapy. In 1948, he described success using movement to treat stress incontinence, which is when physical activity causes urine to leak. He is the namesake of the most famous pelvic floor squeezing exercise, the only one anyone outside the professional field can name, as well as a device for measuring pelvic tone, the Kegel perineometer. The Kegel has saturated popular culture—appearing in postpartum hospital literature, boutique fitness centers, the Kardashians' social feeds, and a litany of hit pieces about Gwyneth Paltrow. A device for tracking them was found in swag bags at the 2017 Academy Awards.

The kind of pelvic floor physical therapy that I have experienced, that Michele practices, can seem like a new specialty because people don't know it exists until they need it badly. However, the knowledge to rehabilitate the pelvic floor predates Kegel by thousands of years.

"Deer exercises," which engaged the pelvic floor to prevent incontinence, were integral to Taoist exercise regimens for over six thousand years. Greeks and Romans toned their pelvic floors during calisthenics routines in public baths and gymnasiums. Indian texts reference pelvic movement. Yoga works with Ashwini Mudra, a practice of tightening the anal sphincter, and Mula Bandha, a Sanskrit term for root lock, a contraction held at the bottom of the pelvis and cervix. When the only thing we know about the pelvic floor is "Do Kegels," we miss out on this ancient wisdom.

There is also a rich recent history of women who have developed methods of comprehensive pelvic floor rehabilitation. In 1912, Minnie Randell, a midwife and physiotherapist, devised a regimen to ready women for childbirth and heal them postpartum. Her method was part of a plan to replace drugs and forceps with natural births at London's St. Thomas Maternity Hospital. The concurrent women's suffrage movement had inspired Randell. She believed that her regimen not only restored health but also helped to empower women more broadly in society.

Randell's physiotherapist colleague Margaret Morris wrote a paper in 1936 describing how vitally important it was for women to engage in "the conscious control of tension and relaxation of the pelvic floor muscles for the prevention and treatment of urinary and faecal incontinence," according to the International Continence Society. She encouraged women to "invert the sphincters ... until it becomes habitual" in repetitions while listening to a Schubert waltz. Function was the goal, not tightness for husbands.

Randell and Morris jointly published an illustrated pregnancy exercise guide that "emphasized breathing, relaxation, conscious training of the pelvic floor muscles, and re-establishing good posture," as researchers put it. By 1940, the St. Thomas Method, or "Training for Childbirth and After," had been implemented in hospitals throughout London and Australia.

Later, in the 1960s and 1970s, physiotherapist Dorothy Mandelstam improved upon pelvic floor exercise, earning her the moniker "Queen of Continence." The Independent described the incontinence specialty as "a Cinderella branch of medicine" where the expectation was merely the "quiet warehousing of destitute and discarded old people" until Mandelstam came along. Her focus differed from her colleagues'. Whereas they applied "the pad, mop and bucket approach … she took a single-minded interest in the causes, alleviation and management of incontinence—long a taboo subject." She published books on pelvic floor maintenance and helped design some of the first pelvic health educational courses. Mandelstam returned dignity to an elderly population of incontinence sufferers who had previously been stigmatized and ignored. She shaped not only pelvic fitness regimens but the pelvic health specialist role we know today.

"We're calling ourselves pelvic health specialists or pelvic health rehabilitation specialists. But I mean, I'm pretty much a vagina physical therapist if I'm going to speak to a layperson about it," says Reardon. Kim Vopni, author of the manual *Your Pelvic Floor*, prefers "vagina coach." The Academy of Pelvic Health Physical Therapy in the United States counts thirty-five hundred therapists, assistants, and students in its ranks. Pelvic health specialists work in hospitals, physical therapy groups, and private practice.

In the tradition of Randell, Morris, and Mandelstam, pelvic specialists have long advocated a holistic approach to restoring the pelvic floor after childbirth. It's curious, then, that the most common prescription today for pelvic floor problems is "Do Kegels." Could it be because of their association with tight vaginas and because they were named for a man?

"A lot of women aren't doing Kegels properly when they just hear that," Reardon told me. "And we're not using those muscles when we need them. Like if you were just lying down in your bed doing Kegels, you actually need to be turning on that muscle when you carry your baby, when you pick something up." The exercise done wrong or done in isolation isn't sufficient because it doesn't integrate into total body function. Most women don't understand how to perform a Kegel, so even if they're trying to do them, they're doing them wrong. A study of one thousand women found 70 percent couldn't do the exercise properly.

Kegels also aren't for everyone. "There is a population of women to support and talk about whose pelvic floors are too tight and have too much tension in them," said the Bay Area pelvic health rehabilitation therapist Alicia Willoughby when I spoke to her. These people have hyper tone, meaning their pelvic floor muscles are rigid to the point that they can't function properly. Kegels could be harmful for these people, who need help loosening, not gripping. "I see women clinically who have tried online programs or baby boot camps and their leaking got worse or they have pain with sex and their pain got worse," Willoughby said. "It's not appropriate for them to do Kegels, but they can learn how to relax their pelvic floor."

FOR ME, HAVING DIASTASIS RECTI MEANT EMBARKING ON A PELVIC floor discovery journey. I've talked to experts, sifted through studies, read books, gone to physical therapy, and, yes, done a bazillion Kegels. I experimented with exercises and therapies, attempting to reintegrate my pelvic floor into how my body moves. I notice that when I feel connected to it, when it's strong, I am less likely to slip into hip or back pain. Orgasm is more accessible and pleasurable. If I can communicate with it when walking, running, or climbing stairs, I can feel an internal boost, an inside hug.

We should know and practice caring for this magician and workhorse as early as menstruation, Vopni explains in her book. Dentists warn that the absence of brushing and flossing, combined with too many saccharine treats, causes cavities. Vopni believes that "female health educators can introduce the concept that daily habits such as posture and the way you go to the toilet, and life events such as childbirth can lead to challenges with your pelvic floor muscles."

A British obstetrician who spent years practicing in India observed that the "active indigenous Indian" lifestyle, which included positions like squatting that maintained optimized pelvic anatomy, made birth easier, while affluent Westerners, who had abandoned those movements, struggled more. Our sedentary existence, pecking at keyboards and craning over devices, doesn't help our ability to give birth. From her Vagina Whisperer platform on Instagram, Reardon evangelizes proper bathroom positioning and breathing. Many of us aren't doing those simple things right. We're forcing and straining. When going to the bathroom, she recommends elevating your feet on a stool, for example, to relax the pelvic floor and exhaling rather than bearing down and straining.

Our bodies move. Parts work in concert. Pelvic health specialists care more about how our pelvic floor supports our daily movements. How do we distribute forces? Moving, breathing, laughing,
coughing, twisting, pooping, sitting, running, jumping, lifting—all
of these activities distribute pressure through the pelvic floor and abdomen. And the goal is to do these activities without leakage or pain.
Pelvic floor muscles shouldn't be straining or pushing to the point
of damage when you're birthing or doing anything else. And pelvic
health isn't something we should be forced to discover on our own,
postpartum, when we're in pain and suffering and desperate for help.
It should be standard, accessible to all.

Obstetrician Alison Stuebe blames the fragmentation of care.
"There are lactation consultants, who are excellent at how the baby's
attaching to the breast. But their training doesn't include mom's mental health or pelvic pain or fourth-degree laceration. There's a urogy-
necologist who might work on the fourth-degree laceration, but she
doesn't know anything about breastfeeding. She's not screening for
depression. Even though having her bottom tear where her rectum
and vagina are connected is pretty depressing," she told me. "Everybody who touches women in this time period should have a shared understanding of what's evidence based, of what's at least expert-opinion
based, about how to deal with problems."

That's certainly part of the struggle. But I blame cultural sexism as
much as, if not more than, healthcare fragmentation. Pair toxic diet
culture with the societal pressure to look like we didn't just give birth,
and we're destined to struggle.

"After we have a baby, it's like our body isn't our own," says pelvic
health specialist Alicia Willoughby. "What is this body and who is it
for? It's for everyone else but me."

CHAPTER 9
BREAST IS BEST

IT'S DAY THREE AFTER I'VE GIVEN BIRTH FOR THE FIRST TIME, AND my nipples are cracked and bleeding. We're all home. The woman who encapsulated my placenta continues to text encouragement. The alternative to it being dried, Vita-mixed, and fashioned into pills—becoming medical waste—made me ache. She is a lactation counselor but not board certified. She recommends I find someone who is, right away, and shares a contact card.

We're feeding and pumping around the clock. An expert is surely an out-of-pocket cost. Besides, how am I going to get there in this state? Visiting the pediatrician feels like scaling a mountain. But we do it. Her weight is low, the doctor tells us. Too low. It's a Friday. We must return Monday for another "weigh-in." We're going to need outside help to pack emergency ounces onto her shrinking frame within forty-eight hours. We go to the lactation consultant, snug in our outerwear. Snow hides the ground, as it has since she was born.

Take off your shirt, Faye instructs in her office, which feels more like a bedroom. She has soft lines around her eyes and warm hands.

Undress the baby, she says.

I do it with Ben's help. We are fragile, exhausted. I'm starving. The whole of my diet seems to dissolve straight into the milk I'm making, proficiently now. The milk we are trying desperately, futilely, to move from my body to hers, without wrecking mine. Faye places our daughter on a scale that resembles a butcher's. I imagine cured meats strung from the ceiling. We'll weigh her before and after she feeds at each breast to determine how many ounces of milk she takes. This will inform us about her efficiency, whether the trouble is with her latch or her suck, or neither, or both. Do what you usually do, Faye says, so she can watch and correct.

This is the good one, I tell her, pointing to my left breast, implying not only that the bad one is on my right but also that there is a moral weight to my chest. Self-consciously, I position the baby on the pillow, her nose even with my nipple, as my online reading instructed. Faye adjusts my daughter's cheek so that her mouth tilts slightly up. I clasp her neck and hair between my thumb and fingers. I pitch her head back and try to scoop her mouth up and over the top of my nipple.

Missed, I mutter to fill the quiet. I want her to know that I know that I did. I proceed to miss again. Several more times. I have the faint memory of water-skiing attempts at summer camp. Trying to rise on the skis before tumbling forward into white spray, water flooding my nose, my brain. A few more goes. Then she latches. I feel a clamp down, the vise of her jaw. I wince.

Hurts? Faye asks. It shouldn't hurt.

Our childbirth class instructor said if breastfeeding hurts then something is wrong. And it still hurts. No matter how many times I hear the idiom. So now what? We try to reposition her so the latch is deeper and I'm not suffering, but without losing our progress. The baby is falling asleep.

Flick the bottom of her foot, she says, and I look at her, confused. Ben and I look at each other. I tap her foot softly. Ben pushes at her toes.

Harder, Faye says. She flicks my daughter's foot, launching a middle finger from her thumb. Hard. It doesn't hurt them, it just wakes them, annoys them out of slumber, she tells us. Wake up, she says.

Later, I will flick a ton. I will flick with gusto. When I want to feed because I'm engorged or running out, or won't be around later. When I'm exhausted and falling asleep myself, but she doesn't want to drink for the precise number of minutes I'm told that she must (nine on the left, twelve on the right). I will flick, flick, flick to instruct her to wake, to drink. But now I'm reluctant. Why are we flicking my tiny, pink, perfect baby?

Turns out, I take to the flicking quickly. I have some frustration to unleash through my fingers onto her foot. Now I'm flicking like a pro. I'm surprised and slightly disturbed when I notice this, but not enough to stop.

How does it stop hurting? I ask. How long until breastfeeding pain ends, is what I mean. Will it ever?

Try the nipple shield, Faye says. You can order them online. They come in different sizes. Order more than one to see what fits. She tells me to stop pumping after feeding, which I've been doing with a chef's focus. You're telling your body, "Twins, twins," she says. A doula told me that everyone's pump talks to them. The same pump can have a different sound and set of words for each woman, each nurser. Mine sounds like "rat poop, rat poop." Over and over.

She prescribes saltwater soaks for my nipples in between feedings. And olive oil, herbaceous and slick, to heal two distinct slashes in my areola that are the source of the burning I feel when she latches. Evening primrose oil should soften clogged ducts, along with rest and water, she says.

She teaches us a series of jaw exercises to open baby's mouth.

She's lazy, I hear from another mother, describing her infant in a movement class I take a few months later. It's not a helpful or true thing to say about a baby, but I can relate to the urge to say it. I've thought it.

Ben does the exercises to her jaw while kneeling on the floor across from me like a shaman. He does as Faye says, fingers massaging circles on her jawbones, running across her upper lip like a mustache, pinching her lips into a "fish face," so they pucker. Then three taps on the mouth repeated three times. This choreography is meant to encourage her mouth to open wide so we can stuff my breast inside. In the hospital, our doula called it a nipple sandwich and said, "Nom nom." I'm desperate and beginning to see spots in the air, I'm so tired. I have dedicated nearly every waking moment since birth to feeding this baby breastmilk. We have a journal full of chicken scratch lists of feeding times, amounts, and session lengths. This was before the influx of apps that both record this and track you.

When I consider that time now, the pain was palpable, but so was the clarity of purpose. I just had to do this one thing. Our society fails so flagrantly at rest, at stillness, at doing nothing, at not producing. I wonder if this is why we struggle to do what is programmed into our biology—feed a newborn and sleep. It was a blessing to learn that feeding is something that can be done *while* sleeping. Doing any other task—laundry, making toast—seemed impossible. Why couldn't I have just stayed in bed with my baby? If we had just laid there together, warm and still, while someone else fed us and kept us relatively clean, could we have learned nursing sooner? Would we have avoided pressure-filled weigh-ins at the (well-meaning!) pediatrician? Voyaging across the city in the cold? The chewed-up nipples, the agony and worry and feelings of failure? I don't think I could stay in bed for a whole day if it were required. The programming always running in the background—that I should be producing, working, achieving something, anything, be it a piece of writing, a load of laundry, or a meal—was too strong. Maybe my nostalgia for having a newborn is really desire for permission and a path to do just one instinctive thing. Even though I couldn't, in the end, do just that.

WHEN I ASKED MOMS WHAT THEY WISHED THEY HAD KNOWN BEfore birth, what would have improved their experiences, breastfeeding came up a lot. Hundreds mentioned it in my survey, and some said it was the single hardest part of becoming a parent. Many were astonished by its difficulty. They had expected "milk to flow like an excretion," in the words of psychologist Donald Winnicott.

"I thought breastfeeding would be like peeing," said Madhu, who had two daughters in New York City. "If you want to make liquid come out of your body, you just do it. It doesn't work that way, and since my mother never breastfed and none of my friends who had gone through motherhood ever talked about it with me, I was very much alone and in the dark."

About 66 percent of my survey respondents used some kind of lactation specialist, but still, overwhelmingly, they had wanted more information and support to breastfeed. That number is likely higher in the general population. Access to lactation consultants varies by geographic availability and income, because most don't accept insurance or Medicaid. However, it's telling that more than half of the group with access still found what they got to be lacking. They wanted to better understand milk supply—how to make more milk, and also how to make less, since oversupply, as it's called, can be painful. Some people had believed that their care providers—nurses, OBGYNs, pediatricians—were the experts who could help and were disappointed to find otherwise. They didn't realize that these specialists don't understand or know how to teach breastfeeding. Some had never heard of the actual breastfeeding experts, lactation consultants. Plenty wanted access to experts sooner or would have used them had they not been so expensive or denied by insurance. Moms wanted to know why initial breastfeeding hurt and how to avoid pain. They wished they had known how time-consuming breastfeeding was.

Two common desires that surfaced in my survey were the need to hear that formula was permissible, that it wasn't poison, and to feel supported and celebrated in the choice to bottle-feed, instead of feeling as if they had failed their first mothering task. New parents wanted to know that it was OK not to breastfeed exclusively, that pumping and bottle-feeding "still counted." They (and, frankly, I) wished they had known the truth: that any amount of breastfeeding, exclusive or just a little, just for comfort, counted. It *all* counts.

As I wrote in the introduction to this book, when I asked moms to choose from a list of adjectives to describe their births (they could select as many or as few as they wanted), a sizable group—fifty-eight people—only chose the descriptor "traumatic." On a question about what kind of information they wished they had at the time, this cohort said they would have liked more information about giving birth itself before they did it. But higher on their list was information about lactation and breastfeeding, the second most popular category of information birthers craved. The first category, at the very top of the list, was information about postpartum mental health, which in many ways is inextricable from lactation and breastfeeding. This finding reified for me the link between birth trauma and the dearth of breastfeeding support. It also made me wonder whether traumatized mothers would have appraised their births differently if they had received breastfeeding information and support—and whether, if breastfeeding were more visible, less stigmatized, more culturally supported, and better understood as part of our daily lives, their stories would have been very different.

Additionally, the moms I surveyed wished they'd experienced less pressure to breastfeed from healthcare professionals. They said that advice, when offered, was often unhelpful or contradictory. Medical staff told them little beyond "Breast is best" or "Keep at it." If new mothers get only such statements, if they're not informed or supported, they likely won't meet their own breastfeeding goals. More than half of women currently don't. Almost no one in the survey who mentioned breastfeeding said it was easy or that they knew a lot about it before doing it. Counterintuitively, American culture ostensibly lionizes yet practically devalues breastfeeding. "Breast is best" has become shorthand for "You're on your own."

Hospital lactation support was abysmal pre-pandemic, and it's grown even worse. In 2020, 18 percent of hospitals reduced their lactation support, and 73 percent discharged mothers and their infants less than forty-eight hours after birth, before most women's milk typically comes in, according to a Centers for Disease Control and Prevention report. Making matters worse, breastfeeding is routinely misrepresented by hospital providers. Doctors and nurses tell many new moms that, based on the size and shape of their breasts and nipples, they likely won't make enough milk—a complete fallacy according to lactation specialist and doula Lauren Archer. "There's lots of different nipple shapes and sizes and each one can feed your baby," she explained.

Meanwhile, some doctors prefer to give and push formula. In 1999, "a majority of pediatricians agreed with or had a neutral opinion about the statement that breastfeeding and formula-feeding [were] equally acceptable methods for feeding infants." And in 2021, Janiya Mitnaul Williams, an international board-certified lactation consultant, recounted how she witnessed NICU physicians pushing formula on preemie babies in recent years because they thought it was superior to human milk, that babies would leave the hospital faster if they drank what science rather than their mothers created.

Underpinning these erroneous assumptions and practices is a suspicion of women's bodies and their capabilities. We trust what we can count—a product, formula, dispensed in ounces. Hospital staff often wrongly believe that babies need to eat immediately after birth, so they ply them with formula, even without asking a mother's permission. Formula exposure in the hospital predicts who will breastfeed beyond discharge, as formula-feeding can interfere with the baby learning to latch onto the breast. This focus on immediate nourishment stems from a misunderstanding of a baby's physiology. Our Bradley Method instructor told us that when a baby is born, her stomach is tiny, the size of a walnut, and already sated at birth—meaning she doesn't need to eat immediately. But healthcare professionals, who are generally not trained in lactation and breastfeeding, rather than assuaging parents' worries, stoke their anxiety. They suggest that their babies could starve. And we readily graft our inherited toxic beliefs about food onto infants just born. They're crying. It must be hunger! Feed them! Then, we arrive at the pediatrician's office and learn they are "underweight," even though most practices use weight benchmarks based on formula-fed babies, not breastfed ones. Because child nutrition researchers are often funded by infant formula companies, and pediatricians use this research to care for babies, growth measurement is entirely misunderstood.

All of this leaves women in the unenviable position of entreating the hospital team to delay formula, seeking out specialists, and traveling *to them* after giving birth. The lack of insurance coverage for lactation specialists, as well as the dearth of Medicaid coverage for postpartum costs, like pelvic floor physical therapy and mental treatments, create even more challenges. And all this is only the preamble to a larger societal scheme to obstruct breastfeeding.

MY MOTHER TOLD ME THAT SHE HAD WANTED TO BREASTFEED BUT couldn't produce enough milk. She spent forever trying to pump an amount that filled a thimble in the New York hospital where I was born. Her dad then dumped out the contents of the small cup into the sink, not realizing what was inside. She felt defeated. She had barely started. Reading between the lines of her experience, and knowing what I know now, she wasn't set up for breastfeeding to work. Those around her didn't support her. Her mother had fed her a bottle. She didn't have a person to model or a group to help.

Little has changed in forty years.

The problem wasn't that she couldn't make milk. She was still in the hospital. Her mature milk hadn't even come in yet. She has never described her struggle like that—she just believed that *she* failed, that *she* couldn't produce. No one, not even her close friend, a nurse, told her that she was already making colostrum, which *is* milk, a potent kind that's small in quantity but dubbed "liquid gold" for its nutrient density, or that her baby needed to be on her chest suckling every sixty to ninety minutes for the mature fluid to start flowing. This knowledge still escapes many moms today.

"It's a demand and supply system," said Jada Shapiro, a lactation counselor and the founder of an on-demand lactation consultant service called Boober. "Your baby has to demand breast milk from your breast by suckling, which triggers hormone production that affects breastmilk production." When a baby suckles at the breast, she stimulates the nipple, the areola, and the breast tissue, which kick-starts the milk-making hormones, like oxytocin and prolactin, Shapiro told me. "This hormone production signals to the brain 'Hey, you need to make more milk,' and then more milk is produced in response."

Babies don't just want their mothers' bodies, they need them. Without the frequent connection and stimulation, Shapiro advises, the milk won't come. "If you restrict and don't do it more frequently than every three hours, almost all people won't make enough milk for their baby," she said. I had birthed and breastfed two kids before anyone told me this, and Shapiro only did so because I was interviewing her for an article I was writing about why we know so little about breastfeeding.

Anyone can become a wedge preventing moms and newborns from successful breastfeeding. I know a woman whose mother-in-law told her she was "selfish and hogging the baby" because of their frequent breastfeeding. Another claimed her daughter-in-law was "forcing the baby to become dependent" on her. This sentiment is present when even well-intentioned people warn moms against becoming a "human pacifier" or suggest that too much contact "spoils the baby." Such comments reflect a misunderstanding about how breastfeeding works and a lack of knowledge about how a baby's frequent exposure to the breast is what enables a new mom's body to make milk. It also serves to police access to women bodies, revealing our society's curdled relationship to them. It presents admission to the breast as a luxury rather than a biological imperative. Maybe a baby's constant access to their mother threatens everyone else's access to her, and to her meeting *their* needs. If she must just do this one thing, make milk, that means she requires a break from doing everything else. But in the US, women get few breaks, if any at all.

Meanwhile, decades after my own mother's breastfeeding angst, women still believe they are failing to breastfeed because their bodies can't produce enough milk. "You don't fret that one day your kidneys will fail or your digestive system won't work. But we consistently doubt that our breasts will perform a basic mammalian function," writes Kimberly Seals Allers in *The Big Letdown*, her book about the forces undermining breastfeeding. "Lactation holds the award for being the one bodily function that we think of as precarious and likely to fail us."

In fact, she says, fewer than 5 percent of women are actually "physically incapable of breastfeeding," though many more are diagnosed with low supply or told that their breasts don't work. But how many of us aren't taught the mechanics and acceptance of breastfeeding, are separated from our babies, and thus believe the low supply farce?

TSEDAYE WALKS INTO THE WELLNESS ROOM CLASPING A BOTTLE OF Evian water. A large lion head tattoo turns on her arm. She's here for breastfeeding education, which she'll put to use very soon. She is thirty-seven weeks pregnant and twenty-four years old, sitting on one side of a large couch. Connie, a lactation specialist at MamaToto Village, a perinatal healthcare and support center for Black women in Washington, DC, sits beneath her on a blue swirl rug, a binder spread across her knees. Sun heats the window and voids the need for an overhead bulb. Connie asks Tsedaye how she's doing, how she's feeling. Tsedaye is excited for her baby to just get here already. She's eager to leave her job at a juvenile detention center, with its toxic environment and punishing schedule. Her shifts run from 2:00 to 11:00 p.m., and she has no set days off.

Connie first asks Tsedaye what kind of support she has at home. Tsedaye lists her boyfriend and her mom, who breastfed four children in infancy, including Tsedaye. Connie applauds this. "Usually, people don't understand breastfeeding, so they speak out of turn," she says. "You come from a breastfeeding family. You're going to be great at this."

Connie ticks off some of breastfeeding's benefits for the baby—boosting the immune system, developing the brain—and others for mom, like hormone regulation, disease prevention, bonding, and cost savings compared to formula. She dispels the myth that breast size dictates milk supply. It's all about the number of milk ducts.

"I was wondering," Tsedaye says, relieved. "Mine didn't really grow."

Connie explains the importance of securing a good latch, describes how a baby's mouth affixes to breast tissue, and points to images of breastfeeding positions on her screen. She clicks to a diagram of different nipple shapes—protruding, inverted, flat. "Flat or inverted may take more patience and time, but there's nothing we can't work with," Connie assures her.

Organizations like MamaToto are critical to addressing racial disparities in breastfeeding. Black women are the least likely group to initiate and maintain breastfeeding and also to plan to do it, according to a 2015 study in the journal *Pediatrics*. They are wrongly blamed for this in hospitals and in research. There is history to consider. Enslaved Black women in the US were once forced to feed their white enslavers' babies before they could feed their own, leaving their children undernourished and disease prone. This fanned the stereotype that Black children were weaker and less vital than white ones. Black procreation sustained the institution of slavery while Black breastfeeding sustained the enslavers, according to the sociologist Dorothy Roberts. Freed Blacks moved away from wet nursing and breastfeeding with the advent and popularization of formula during the Great Depression. This bitter history has implications for Black women breastfeeding in America today.

Another profound barrier to breastfeeding for Black people is what Mitnaul Williams calls the mirror-mirror effect. "People of color tend to receive messages about health better from other people who look like them" because of deep mistrust of the medical establishment, she said in an interview. Far too few lactation consultants and advocates identify as Black, something she is working to change.

The International Board of Lactation Consultant Examiners is the global organization that trains and certifies lactation specialists, who, once they complete coursework and pass an exam, can practice anywhere in the world. While those who take the test divulge their racial and ethnic backgrounds, the organization doesn't share that data publicly, Mitnaul Williams said. She and colleagues estimate that less than 2 percent of all IBCLCs (International Board Certified Lactation Consultants) are Black or African American.

Racist stereotypes about lack of education, ability, and laziness persist and coalesce to fault Black women for low breastfeeding rates, when in fact the paucity of support and resources is to blame, according to Thérèse Cator, founder of the community

Embodied Black Girl. For instance, Black women are the most likely group to get formula in the hospital. Providers don't trust them to make milk or to breastfeed successfully. And as mentioned above, formula exposure in the hospital predicts who will breastfeed beyond discharge. In that context, Black lactation specialists teaching and supporting Black breastfeeding, like those at Mama-Toto, are doing work that's as radical as it is essential.

Thanks to MamaToto, Tsedaye already knows that breastfeeding is a round-the-clock job. She wants the baby with her immediately after birth so that her body will produce the oxytocin and prolactin hormones that make milk flow. Written into her birth plan are skin-to-skin, waiting to clamp the umbilical cord, and keeping her baby with her. Connie isn't going anywhere either. When Tsedaye's baby arrives and she has questions or needs breastfeeding support, Connie can help.

Sitting in the room with them, I am jealous. I wonder if intimate instruction like this during pregnancy could have made nursing initiation easier for me in the weeks and months after I gave birth for the first time. Instead, the hospital lactation consultant I phoned never called back or came to my room. Nurses assured me I could see her in a class she taught. It was less a class than a screening—disheveled mothers in hospitals gowns watching a video in a converted closet, our babies beside us in clear plastic bassinets. In the video, a hand stroked a breast to classical music. There was no head or lower body. After very few strokes, milk spewed as from a fire hose. We stared like cartoon characters, collecting stretched jaws from the floor. The only liquid my body was making was tears. The crying seemed to be contagious. I got up and left.

Once I could nurse without guards or Ben squatting in front of us to play percussion on our daughter's face, other challenges arose. My body produced an oversupply of milk, repeatedly engorging my breasts to the point of pain. I fought infections like mastitis and thrush, and clogged ducts were at times more agonizing than birth itself. One night I awoke with such a massive, painful clog that even gravity on my chest from standing up was unbearable. After applying hot and cool compresses (I couldn't tell which, if either, was effective), I dropped to all fours and shook with sobs so loud that I woke my husband. He applied pressure, pushing the knot toward my nipple, milking me, as I was in too much agony to do it myself. This wasn't taught in my birthing class. I didn't know any of this would occur. Maybe if someone had told me, I still would have experienced it all the same way. But maybe not.

In birthing class, we positioned plastic dolls at chest level on our sweaters. I had other things to worry about—not tearing, buying the right stuff. I made spreadsheets comparing different brands of strollers, cribs, and monitors. I imagined there wasn't much to learn about breastfeeding until one actually had a baby to do it with. Later, after having probably my thirtieth clogged duct over the course of nursing three kids, a midwife told me that the best medicine wasn't complicated. She recommended water and rest. She said that clogs are your body's way of telling you to slow down, that you're doing too much.

In July 2021, I drove to a book event for the parenting expert Emily Oster. As I parked my car, I noticed a man stepping out of a white Tesla, clutching her new book in his hand. I had expected nearly all women attendees, as is common at parenting talks. But there he was, the only man, save two staffers in a group of a dozen women.

He was the first attendee to speak. He was wearing sunglasses because we were outside, but the parts of his face not hidden behind them grew violet as his voice wobbled. His wife had worked so hard at trying to breastfeed. Killed herself to do it. But it hadn't gone well. Their pediatrician, whom they sought out for help, offered no consolation. "Breast is best," the doctor had said, which made them, him, his wife, feel like failures. Then he began to cry or to fight off crying, some combination, while self-consciously name-checking the tears and wondering aloud why they needed to flow, as if questioning would stop them. I felt for him and knew that strategy wouldn't work for me.

It was good that we had your book, he said, voice hoarse. Because we learned that it wouldn't kill our kid if she didn't breastfeed. It was fine. One day we just gave the baby some formula, and the baby was happy, and we were happy and realized this was even a little bit fun.

Oster smiled compassionately. His story, while tender, was no anomaly for her. She gets lots of emails from dads about this very thing. One stood out in her mind: the dad who wrote her to say that his wife was failing to breastfeed and that it was destroying their family. He added that his wife was an Emily Oster devotee. Could Emily just tell her that it was OK to stop? The dad believed that if she could just communicate to his wife directly that quitting breastfeeding was OK, she would listen, and their family could then vault over this stumbling block. She just needed permission from an expert. One who had synthesized *the studies*. And not just any expert but a famous one.

How did we get here?

A popular, seemingly feminist argument today is that women feel too much pressure to breastfeed. I first took note of it in August 2021 when my mom texted me a screenshot of a full-page advertisement in the *New York Times* that appeared at the start of National Breastfeeding Month.

"How is breastfeeding going?" asks the ad, but the word *breast* is crossed out. Four parents' portraits fill the page. One mother stands on a breast pump. "Don't assume I can do it all," reads the caption beneath her. Another bottle feeds a baby while topless. "Don't assume my breasts can make milk," hers says. A third hugs four children ("Don't assume breast was best for my entire family"), and a fourth, Tan France of the *Queer Eye* reboot, clasps a photo of his child in utero: "Don't assume I want to feed my baby donor breastmilk." In large print below the parents, the ad says, "Nearly 75% of U.S. parents will turn to formula within the first 6 months. So why are we ashamed to talk about it? It's time to evolve the conversation. We'll start."

It was clear that the conversation was about infant feeding, but I wondered who, exactly, was evolving it. And to where? I noticed the name "Bobbie" written just below the text. When I Googled it, I learned that Bobbie was an organic baby formula company that had launched a few months earlier. I felt warm with anger, complained to Ben. Could he believe this? He shrugged. Because, as he told me later, a formula company taking out a full-page *New York Times* ad to trash breastfeeding is highly believable!

Feminist anti-breastfeeding rhetoric is omnipresent. "The breast is best movement" has become a target, "creating anxiety for new mothers who struggle physically, mentally or emotionally with the sometimes painful and always time-consuming task of breastfeeding," *Time* magazine declared in 2021. "Breast is best left me feeling broken, ashamed, overwhelmed and exhausted," wrote Kristen Thompson in the Canadian website *Today's Parent*. "Those feelings, echoed by thousands of other women who struggle with nursing, explain the growing backlash against the exclusive-breastfeeding movement, even among people who agree with it in principle," she observes, arguing that now is the time "to retire the phrase 'breast is best' once and for all."

Covid has kindled infinite cultural problems, including, apparently, intensifying the pressure to breastfeed. Covid-fighting antibodies occur in human milk, suggesting protection for babies who drink it. This is great news (though it shouldn't surprise us, as one of breastmilk's known amazing qualities is fighting disease), but according to *Time*, it's also handicapping moms. "Covid-19 Is Making New Moms Feel Even More Pressure to Breastfeed" is the title of a 2021 article.

At first, I couldn't understand why this framing vexed me. *I* struggled to breastfeed. I pressured myself to continue, when I was failing, as it grew increasingly sadistic. Like these other moms, I had experienced the shame and exhaustion. Furthermore, I believe people should decide for themselves how to use their bodies and what to feed their kids.

Eventually I realized that the argument grates because it conceals the real problem and who is at fault. The problem isn't the pressure on moms to breastfeed and the solution isn't formula. The culprit is a wholesale failure of hospitals, the healthcare system, workplaces, and communities to support caregiving and motherhood. The beginning of a solution is demanding accountability from them.

Allers, *The Big Letdown* author, says that people don't breastfeed, cultures do. And our culture, largely, doesn't. Paternalistic institutions ensure that we struggle or quit, then blame us for stopping. You can't breastfeed if you aren't being cared for as you recuperate and heal from birth. If you are separated from your baby because of others' needs or the mandates of your workplace. If you're undernourished or don't feel safe and well. You also likely can't and won't breastfeed if it's unclear how to do it, if no one supports you through what can be a bewildering journey full of shitshows and pitfalls. And who would want to breastfeed when we're taught that it isn't for our benefit—that it's a pointless sacrifice we make for others?

We should absolutely validate the anxiety parents feel about breastfeeding, but if we stop there, we're only individualizing a universal experience and ensuring that parents internalize blame. This is exactly how internalized sexism and racism work: women and Black people are hoodwinked into believing that societal and structural problems are individual ones. Close to 90 percent of people who give birth attempt breastfeeding. The desire is there. What's not is the support, the community, and the care. Ours is not a breastfeeding culture.

And then there's the profit motive—the lack of one for breastfeeding and the billions of dollars spent on formula. Companies ensure formula leaves with you in your hospital bag or arrives unsolicited in a giant box on your doorstep, as was the case for me before I even brought my baby home. The federal government subsidizes our breast pumps (thanks, Obama), but not because our country cares for families—rather, so you'll return to work. Some 25 percent of women return to work just ten days after their babies are born. Rather than supplying adequate paid leave, we get machines to use alone in closets. Those of us lucky enough to scrounge some maternity leave might be able to establish breastfeeding during that time, but then we're back to our jobs and the weaning commences whether we want it to or not. This is what happened to me with two of my kids. I had to return to work and thought the pump would keep us breastfeeding when it was actually an offramp to stopping sooner than we might have liked. We're nudged to fail under the guise of being accommodated.

Nursing in the US is lonely work. Moms breastfeed shrouded in fabric, in rooms with closed doors. When you pull out your boob, people look away, they leave the room. This happened to me all the time—everywhere from public spaces to my parents' house.

We're told infant feeding is individual choice, not societal concern. "Women not meeting breastfeeding goals is presented as individual failure. That is such a lie. It's such a fiction," said Katie Hinde, a lactation researcher and professor of evolutionary biology at Arizona State University. Hinde gave a TED talk that revealed we know more about the composition of a tomato than we do about human milk. In 2007, the National Institutes of Health announced that it would dedicate $115 million and five years to studying three hundred human specimens—blood, skin, amniotic fluid, saliva, snot, feces, and more—to create a library of the body's colonies of microbes, vitally important to human health. Perplexingly, it omitted breastmilk.

The sizable profit gleaned from this gaslighting can't be ignored. And the problem is compounded and magnified by national marketing campaigns that use National Breastfeeding Month to "evolve the conversation around infant feeding," when they are actually co-opting a cultural and policy failure to hawk a product. "It's a very big industry that wants to just not have women figure out, if they want to, how to be able to breastfeed," said Kavita Patel. Before she was a hospital executive, she served as a healthcare policy director in the Obama administration and negotiated breastfeeding accommodations in the 2010 Affordable Care Act. Patel told me that when the American Association of Insurance Plans surveyed their member companies' own offerings, they found that only 10 percent of the plans offered any lactation service coverage.

"I didn't think it was a big deal to include lactation services," she told me. "I'm like, 'Who is going to argue with me?' There's nothing to argue about. Well, the formula lobby is basically as big as the agriculture lobby."

Patel felt that companies like Nestlé were trying to convince the administration that covering lactation services was bad for women. "They brought in moms who had the saddest stories—moms of babies who had died because they couldn't breastfeed. And there is this cultural story, you know: breast is best. And I said, 'I understand all that, and it's terrible what happened to these women. But that doesn't mean that a woman with plugged ducts or something legitimate that requires some help should not get that help. That's crazy.'"

Patel also argued for virtual visits with lactation consultants.

"If you've got a little baby, there's no reason for you to have to go schlep into an office. You should just be able to do this over video," she explained. "I didn't win that battle. Insurers wouldn't pay for that. The fundamental argument is they did not want to pay for something they didn't have to. And that was it. They didn't feel like they had to."

Thanks to Patel and other officials, the Affordable Care Act mandates that plans cover lactation services. Congress didn't specify how may visits, or over what period of time, because, as Patel put it, lawmakers shouldn't dictate how medicine is practiced. As a government official she understood policy, but as a physician she also understood what goes on in treatment rooms. Insurance companies tried to pressure her, claiming that OBGYNs should be on the hook for providing lactation services, but she corrected them: "That's not what they do." Incredibly, it wasn't until 2016 that ACOG formally included lactation as part of its clinical practice recommendations. "Nobody gets training on breastfeeding in medical school," Patel said. "Maybe they should."

Meanwhile, the other doctor whom women see in the days and weeks after birth is the pediatrician. No surprise, then, that the American Academy of Pediatrics (AAP) was first created in 1930 to distribute formula. The thirty-five physicians who founded it saw formula as the revolution that it was for sick or orphaned infants. However, to become the multi-billion-dollar industry it is today, formula needed a wider audience. It found one by demonizing breastfeeding and convincing women that they couldn't make milk.

Only later did the AAP become a child healthcare advocacy organization. However, it's still bound up with and pushing formula. Three of the top donors to the AAP's corporate fund are Nestlé, Abbott, and Reckitt Mead Johnson, the largest infant formula companies.

On a hot summer day in 1956, Mary White and Marian Tompson sat shaded beneath a tree in a suburban Chicago park, chatting and breastfeeding their babies. Other mothers warmed and cooled milk bottles, wrestling them into children's mouths. Soon, curious mothers approached the two under the tree.

"I wanted to nurse my baby, but my doctor told me I didn't have enough milk," said one. Another woman's mother-in-law told her the baby was starving, obviously, based on how frequently he wanted to nurse. A third thought her baby had "lost interest," when she supplemented with formula. Their messages unified into a mantra: I tried to breastfeed, but I couldn't. White and Tompson could relate. The children they were nursing beneath that tree weren't their first. The incident imprinted onto Tompson. She realized two things: women were settling for bottle-feeding as a "second choice," and their struggles could have been overcome with "a little information and a lot of encouragement."

This is a truncated origin story of America's oldest breastfeeding support organization. Naming it was tricky. Newspapers, the natural space to advertise meetings, wouldn't print the word *breast*, considering it lewd. Edwina Froehlich, a founding mother, joked that "in those days you didn't mention 'breast' in print unless you were talking about Jean Harlow."

The founders resisted calling it a nursing group, lest it be confused with a professional organization for nurses. Their husbands suggested "Milk Maids" or "Busty Broads." But the founders' Catholic ties ultimately helped them choose. They named themselves for a statue of Mary nursing Jesus: *Nuestra Señora de la Leche y Buen Parto*, which translates to "Our lady of milk and good birth." The statue symbolized the flavor of motherhood the group was trying to elevate and sell to members. It still stands inside a moss-covered chapel in St. Augustine, Florida, a stop on the town's historic sites trolley tour.

Tompson, White, and five friends held their first La Leche League meeting in October 1956 at White's Franklin Park home. White's physician husband served as a medical advisor. Tompson borrowed the support group meeting style from the Christian Family Movement, a religious community working for social justice. The La Leche League meeting structure devised in the late 1950s, in which a leader guides a conversation between mothers about breastfeeding and motherhood, is virtually unchanged today. The leader is an experienced breast-feeder. However, leader is a misnomer. She's more like a facilitator, moving the conversation along in the group—but her decentralized authority is exactly what allows the collective to thrive. Every attendee is there both to teach and to learn. The leader offers snippets from her own experience, but she mostly speaks to validate others, not to instruct them.

It's important to understand how radical this was at the time. In 1956, just a third of babies drank breastmilk after hospital discharge. Formula was routine, believed to be superior because it was scientific. Birth itself was grisly—"twilight sleep" drugs knocked women unconscious and instigated temporary waist-down paralysis. "No more devastating image could be invented for the bondage of woman: sheeted, supine, drugged, her wrists strapped down and her legs in stirrups, at the very moment when she is bringing life into the world," observed Adrienne Rich of birth in this era. It's an understatement to say La Leche League attendees were outliers in believing they could feed babies with their bodies.

Their determination was a product of their privilege. White, upper-middle-class, Catholic women could center their struggles and pursue individualism through motherhood in a way that wasn't available to all women. La Leche League was "a place of affirmation," wrote author and academic Chris Bobel in her qualitative analysis of groups in southern Wisconsin. It proffered a brand of radical feminism through breastfeeding. "The league could be credited for its role in rejecting sexist portrayals of women's bodies as primarily objects for male consumption," Bobel explained. "By asserting the natural and functional role of a woman's breasts as providers of nourishment, a woman's body resists sexualized male exploitation," she continued. One of her study participants, Rachel, described her changed relationship to her breasts: "I view my breasts differently since I started breast-feeding.

There is so much more to them. I learned that they are not just something to be harassed about. Breastfeeding instills appreciation of
your body. It forces you to listen to your body." Natural childbirth
and breastfeeding swayed La Leche members to "reclaim control of
their bodies." Bobel cites research that those who breastfeed appreciate their own bodies because they do it and that breastfed babies are
more likely to grow up to view breasts as sources of comfort rather
than the fetish objects they've become, in part because formula feeding is the norm.

In 1957, the group published what would become its manual, a
loose-leaf guide of stories and learnings from the founders and their
children. The second hardcover edition of *The Womanly Art of Breastfeeding* has undergone twenty-nine printings and sold more than 1.1
million copies. La Leche's efforts spread internationally, and it part-
nered with UNICEF, the World Health Organization (WHO), and
the Special Supplemental Nutrition Program for Women, Infants, and
Children to bring its model and message to more women beyond the
group's white, suburban, Catholic founders.

Hewing to religion and its traditionalist notions of women's roles
in the 1970s, the group was largely left out of or opposed to the major
feminist happenings of the day. It refused to publicly support abortion rights and continued to use religious language in its publications.
When women went to work in greater numbers, La Leche refused to
back them. Although supporting women who struggled against their
employers to breastfeed or pump milk at work was a natural avenue
for the group to expand both its advocacy and its visibility, its leaders
declined. Instead, they held fast to the notion that mothers and infants belonged together, not separated by work or anything else. Thus,
throughout the 1980s, La Leche sat by and watched (and grumbled),
losing ground with this cultural transition and the women at its fore-
front. Ironically, many women who went to work still wanted to nurse,
and they needed a champion. La Leche League wasn't it.

I didn't know any of this history when I walked through the door
of a garden apartment in Brooklyn to attend my first La Leche League
meeting more than sixty years after the group's founding, *The Daily*

in my earbuds and a seven-week-old smushed to my chest. I had first heard of La Leche League years earlier, shortly before the birth of my first child. The instructor in my birth education class recommended it. She sent dates for La Leche League meetings to our small group of three expecting couples, but it seemed strange to attend one without a baby. It didn't register as something I would need, something for me. When I needed breastfeeding help with my first child, I looked up local meetings, but it was just after New Year's, and they wouldn't resume for weeks. I had the vague thought that any organization dedicated to teaching and supporting breastfeeding must be feminist, but then wondered why I hadn't heard of others in my progressive community attending. I cringed at the thought of removing my shirt in a room full of strangers (but laugh at that now). I was viewing birth from an individual mindset, not a collective one. I wasn't aware that my knowing nothing about breastfeeding didn't mean that my presence wasn't useful to others. Even as a pregnant, childless person at La Leche League, I could have offered encouragement.

It only felt doable for me to attend with my third child once we had successfully initiated breastfeeding and I was looking for something to do with him during the day. As I sat on a firm couch at that first gathering, I realized I was looking for a group of people going through exactly what I was going through in that moment, a community of other mothers who cared about this thing no one else did.

La Leche League meetings are the only environment where I receive full-on breastfeeding cheerleading and support. They prove that helping people breastfeed doesn't have to be expensive or complicated. It's just a choice we can make. For me, La Leche League was less a location to learn to breastfeed than a place to help me keep going. I still attend a meeting for parents breastfeeding toddlers. We are both students and teachers. There are always tears. The space can hold them. The leader echoes what attendees say and reflects their statements back to them, in a manner not unlike therapy.

I'M NOT SUPPOSED TO SAY THAT I BREASTFEED MY THREE-YEAR-old because I like it. I'm supposed to say he needs it, he won't quit. That I'm prostrating myself, surrendering my body and my time on the altar of attentive, attached motherhood. He enjoys it too, of course. He usually asks. I rarely offer. I don't think I'd make him if he didn't want to. Some days go by, and we don't do it. As I write this, in the summer of 2022, we do it a couple of times a day. More on weekends or when he's hurt, sick, or just wants to. It's his comfort, his lodestar. It also feels good. To me. It eases my anxiety. It fills me with love. It is sentimental, sensory, and sensual. Even more special since I didn't do it this long with my other kids.

One day it hits me that my son and I are nearing "mom enough" territory. You may remember the *Time* magazine cover of a mother nursing a large toddler while he stands on a chair. I worked at a rival magazine when it came out in 2012 and recall standing with a group of editors in a semicircle around the early edition. We stared, tensed our shoulders. I stood quietly, sifting my feelings into an opinion. Was it right or was it wrong? I was married, childless, not yet thirty. It was startling to confront breastfeeding alongside respected senior colleagues, especially since I had hardly thought about it before. Also, as a self-identified feminist, shouldn't my default be loud, unwavering support?

Years earlier, back in college, I had sat beside a mother on an airplane who asked if I minded as she nursed her toddler during the flight. I said no, of course not. She schooled me on benefits for babies and the politics of nursing in public. I nodded, tried not to look. I remember feeling a blend of sympathy and discomfort as I tried on a mother identity in my mind—imagined whether or not I would ever breastfeed in that way, in public, a kid old enough to run, to feed himself, to speak multiclause sentences. It was my first exposure to a person nursing in front of me. I would barely experience that again until my own baby was at my breast.

On the *Time* cover, twenty-six-year-old mother Jamie Lynne Grumet stands with one hand on her hip, her navy tank top pulled down. Her other hand scoops her three-year-old son, who stands on a tiny chair in army fatigues and sneakers, into a half-hug. His mouth around her nipple, as he nurses, looking askew at the camera. The image invoked outrage. Thin, white, and blonde, Grumet was a woman America is accustomed to processing as a sex object marketing something, not a maternal figure nourishing her kid. Critics charged her with scarring or psychologically damaging him, revealing how our society equates feeding with bottles, not breasts. The magazine article wasn't even about breastfeeding. It focused on attachment parenting, an empty label that appears to exist to pit moms against each other and sell them stuff. The cover line both taunts and insults: "Are You Mom Enough?"

The picture was a Rorschach test asking, To whom do breasts belong and what are they for? "I liked the idea of having the kid standing up to underline the point that this was an uncommon situation," said photographer Martin Schoeller, who captured the image. The point appeared to be that the mom was hot, the kid was old, and we, the viewers, were implicated voyeurs in the pair's taboo behavior.

Another photo of Grumet nursing in a seated position appears inside the magazine. Looking at it now, I'm struck by how much they look like my son and me nursing. My son is large—in the ninety-ninth percentile for weight and height—so when he sits in my lap, his legs extend off the furniture, though he tries to curl them to become the smaller baby he once was. He squeals, then smushes my breast to his face with both hands, sometimes sucking and looking at me, sometimes drinking while humming a song or driving a matchbox car along my collarbone.

Our culture has a skewed relationship to breasts. In America, breast augmentation is the second most popular plastic surgery. Entire ad campaigns rest on cleavage. "Bare breasts are welcome if they are used to sell objects, including women's own bodies, but not if there are babies or children attached to them," explains B. J. Woodstein in *The Portrayal of Breastfeeding in Literature*. This becomes truer the more person-like babies become.

I heard about a woman whose pastor asked her not to breastfeed in church because "it caused an older gentleman to have unhealthy thoughts." A male acquaintance made a grotesque comparison: nursing was like him "having his nuts hanging out for everyone to see." I heard about a stranger telling a woman, while she was breastfeeding, that "people who breastfeed just want to show off their tits." These statements reveal an unhealthy fixation on breasts, imagining breastfeeding as sexualized, selfish, and lewd. Comments like these expose their speakers as sexist. They don't characterize breastfeeding.

Florence Williams, author of *Breasts: A Natural and Unnatural History*, muses that breasts (the only organ without its own medical specialty, she notes) were not always universally perceived to be sexual—time, place, and culture molded this. She references tribes and societies in which women live bare chested to breastfeed with ease and cites the statues and paintings of women's breasts and breastfeeding displayed prominently and often throughout Europe as proof that breasts can be celebrated for function and maternal love.

Women in Mali were aghast when anthropologist Katherine Dettwyler told them that Americans lusted after breasts. "You mean men act like babies," they replied, through laughter. Historians speculate that the spread of Christianity and its dictates about female modesty sexualized breasts and that attendant Puritan beliefs actually engendered breast fetishization.

While breastfeeding activists have long pushed to disconnect sex from breasts and accentuate their kid-feeding purpose, research suggests that pleasure and breastfeeding are purposely intertwined. Nipple stimulation can feel good. Some of us don't need the science to prove that, but it exists. Barry Komisaruk, a psychology professor at Rutgers who studies sex, found that stimulating both women's and men's nipples activated the same brain regions as touching their genitals. This could help explain why nipple touching is erotic, he theorized, and why breastfeeding feels good. "Maybe that's an iconoclastic idea that nursing shouldn't be erotically pleasurable," he told writer Jennifer Grayson in her book *Unlatched*. "But what's pleasurable is propagated and maintained in the species. I mean, if it were aversive, then maybe women wouldn't want to nurse." Sex feels good, so we procreate. Breastfeeding is pleasurable, so we feed our kids.

We should be able to hold both ideas: breasts are sources of nour-ishment and comfort for children and eroticism for ourselves. Touch-ing them feels good. Breastfeeding is pleasurable for breastfeeders. We can enjoy our own breasts. We can get off on them—alone, with others. They are also a parenting tool. "There are cultures where breasts are viewed as both sexy and maternal—where women are not classified as mothers or whores, but as sexy and maternal at the same time," Dettwyler said. "It is clearly possible to view breasts as sex ob-jects and still have a totally breastfeeding culture—India does it. But that is not how the United States has gone."

I've heard women describe having had intense orgasms while breast-feeding. "My turn," says my husband, pushing his stubbled cheek next to our son's, as the three-year-old not only sucks my breast but holds it in both hands. He grips tighter, as if his attachment is threatened, even though it's a joke. We all laugh. We know it's a joke. And it's not.

THE "BREAST IS BEST" DRUMBEAT SUGGESTS THAT BREASTFEEDING initiation and breastfeeding as nutrition are the whole of what breast-feeding is. The bulk of research devoted to understanding breastfeeding is on the nutritive benefits during the first six months to the first year of an infant's life. We know some things about how babies benefit when breastmilk is the exclusive first food. But nutritive early breastfeeding isn't the only kind. While bodies like the WHO recommend breast-feeding babies for two years, we know practically nothing about breast-feeding beyond that point because we don't study it. Many people do in fact breastfeed beyond two years. In some cultures, it's common to breastfeed until adult molars come in, at around five or six years old.

How long did you breastfeed? I ask my friend Rachel.

We had kids around the same time—my first, her only—but I re-member that she continued breastfeeding long after I had stopped. She posted photos of her child breastfeeding on social media that I'd heart. I didn't really notice when the photos ceased. Life continued.

You don't want to know, she tells me, leaning in, handing me a glass of champagne. We are at a bar. Ensconced by dark wood.

I do! I say with more emphasis than necessary. I tell her I'm still breastfeeding my three-year-old. No signs of stopping. I don't have many people I can talk to about going this long. Far beyond when you're the food. They have other food now.

You can't talk about it, she continues. I did at first, but my kid got older, and I stopped. People think you're crazy. Maybe I was crazy.

So much shame, I muse.

How did you stop? I ask. When?

Everyone asks this. I hate being asked this. The subtext is, When is enough? Doing this act with your body and your child who can walk and talk. Most people more closely associate something that looks like this with sex, with porn. With the erotic. With adults.

When her daughter was six, Rachel just told her it was the last time. And it was.

We know very little about the benefits of extended breastfeeding. Breastmilk is a live substance, ever-changing, delicious, preventing diseases known and unknown. There's a nutritional reason to continue. That breastfeeding is a movement program is less obvious. As biomechanist Katy Bowman told me, "We see movement as medicine for many things. We haven't thought of breastfeeding as an early infant movement program, a foundation of things to come. If indeed breastfeeding is this amazing natural movement training program for jaw, future teeth, chewing strength, and breathing capabilities, then we have to [reevaluate] our timelines for recommending breastfeeding." Bowman suggests that breastfeeding should last longer than it currently does.

Calling it "extended" breastfeeding makes it an oddity—past what is expected, normal, or reasonable. Beyond its purpose as a product that can be extracted in private, fed to your kid by anyone. I heard the arbitrary response that breastfeeding is perverse after three months. A pediatrician and an obstetrician separately told me that breastfeeding beyond six months is "just for the mom."

It's almost certainly not. But so what if it is? It's curious that when the act tips from benefiting babies to benefiting mothers, the censure flares. Breastfeeding's rewards for moms are manifold and significant—steep reduction in cancers of the breast and ovaries, reduced osteoporosis and postpartum depression and anxiety, improved mood. You get an oxytocin hit every time too. It feels good in your head, in your body. It creates a closeness with your kid. A language you can use to be with each other. Benefits aside, a mom's desire to do it should be reason enough. By the time breastfeeding moves beyond absolute necessity, beyond engorgement, spraying milk everywhere and soaking clothes, by the time it becomes pleasurable, anxiety diffusing, a bonding tool, that's when you're urged to quit, to move on. Because doing it "for the mom" is wrong.

Some women are forced into this choice. In 1991, the department of social services in Syracuse, New York, took white single mom Denise's daughter away from her for a year after she expressed concern that she was becoming sexually aroused while breastfeeding. Denise had called a volunteer center for help reaching La Leche League—she needed support, encouragement, other women to normalize her experience. Instead, the person she spoke to alerted a rape crisis center, which called a child abuse hotline. Denise was charged with child endangerment and sex abuse and spent a night in jail. Because of a constellation of ignorance, miscommunication, and red tape, her daughter went into foster care. Even though the charges were eventually dropped, this horrific ordeal is an example of the punishment that can come from our society's misunderstanding of what breastfeeding is and who it is for.

Some partners try to mandate the end of breastfeeding. I joined a Zoom La Leche League meeting recently and met a mom, Joanna. She was weepy about ceasing breastfeeding her daughter before they both were ready. Her voice shook, and her forehead puckered as she spoke of it. She was separating from her husband, the child's father, and was "court-ordered" to stop breastfeeding, presumably because he believed breastfeeding was interfering with his relationship with his child. A lawyer I spoke to told me this tactic is common in child custody cases involving mothers and their nurslings. Partners can use the stigma, already baked into society, as a wedge.

NO ONE SHOULD FEEL SHAME ABOUT THEIR FEEDING CHOICES—
everyone should make decisions that suit their body and family. But
we're not choosing. "The onus for supporting breastfeeding productively
needs to be on employers, legislators, and clinicians to provide support
and financial flexibility that allows our society to facilitate more babies
and mothers getting the best start," Hinde explained. When we live in
a society that stymies breastfeeding, we don't choose. It chooses for us.

La Leche League leader Anne January described breastfeeding to
me as a parenting framework. I really appreciate the idea that my kid
comes to nurse for comfort, to regroup, as a pick-me-up or expression
of love. But most women won't experience this. For most women, what
feels like a natural conclusion to breastfeeding is actually a confluence
of forces masquerading as support. As concern for mom, even—her
body, space, money, and time. I thought I chose to stop with my older
children, but I didn't. The pump and the bottle were presented as
paths to freedom. Instead, they were the beginning of the end.

Now I look forward to returning home at the end of the day to nurse
my three-year-old. It's when my shoulders lower, I exhale deeply,
snuggle him close, put my feet up, look in his eyes, and get a shot of
oxytocin. To nurse is to be flooded with love. Sometimes I wonder
why we must find verbal substitutes for what our bodies know and can
communicate. Soothing is a language.

We play, I tickle his back, he hums a song. It's a universe away from
the existential chaos of cracked nipples, feeding anxiety, and being
milked by my partner—though I'm grateful for that part. It is my journey too. But I'm glad to be along the road apiece, where breastfeeding
is a practice that feels gratifying, pleasurable, and anxiety reducing. I
feel loved, and so does my son. We create this space for love and give it
to each other with our bodies. But you can't say that. I'm not supposed
to want this. I'm not supposed to breastfeed unless my milk is food.
It's permissible so long as the act is productized. The longer I do it and
enjoy it, the more radical it feels. I'm saying I can do with my body
what I want.

CHAPTER 10

GOOD ENOUGH

THERE IS NO DIAGNOSTIC CODE FOR POSTPARTUM ANXIETY DISOR-der, my therapist—my first who wasn't a childhood punishment—tells me. Health insurance requires a code to cover treatment, she says on the phone. During our first forty-five-minute session, she will search for a diagnosis to pin on me. Whether or not there is one.

I ask her why it's important to diagnose. I am resistant.

She says sometimes patients benefit from having an actual diagnosis if there is one. Sometimes one doesn't exist. More often, one does.

There *is* a diagnostic code for generalized anxiety disorder, she says, when we meet. We can give me that.

Is that what I have?

We don't know yet, she says, but it sounds closest to what you're describing.

I will submit this to my insurer in hopes that it will cover some portion of the therapy costs.

The word "patient" rankles. In my head I had tried "client," but a therapist is not an architect, a travel agent, a gig employer. "Client" is not right. I have never been diagnosed with a mental health disorder. Before today, if someone had asked me whether or not I struggled with mental health, I would have tried hard to project empathy for those who suffer, I would have forgotten how often I use the term PTSD for things that aren't, and then I would have said, Me personally? No.

Today, I'm getting generalized anxiety disorder whether I have it or not.

I've gone from pregnant to not pregnant. The hormones have re-shuffled. It began with heart palpitations. Gone mush in the brain, I googled things like "heart racing" and "fast heartbeat." Whatever I'm experiencing seems to have both an interiority and a physical qual-ity. A jar of small beads endlessly spilling inside my chest cavity. This feeling ignites with my infant's shrieks, which sound derived from a horror film and garner stares in public.

I wonder why this is happening now, after my third birth. I didn't remember feeling this sensation after the previous two. In fact, before the birth, I had been researching and writing about birth trauma and postpartum PTSD. I had spoken to so many moms who experienced these things and experts who treated them. I read that "postnatal dis-tress" plagues almost half of new mothers and a quarter of fathers. I bet it's more; that study is a decade old. I also don't know how they define distress. My dictionary calls it "extreme anxiety, sorrow, or pain." I tell my therapist that I had thought that all my reporting, my knowledge gathering, would shield me from experiencing it. I've tried to shield myself with researching and reporting on many subjects in my career—rape, abortion, C-section, abuse. I thought if I could learn enough about a thing that I could prevent it from afflicting me. Even if it already had.

I'm also surprised because I know how closely connected postpar-tum mental illness is to familial and societal presence. I know that cre-ating ritual and strong support is protective against depression and distress. We see this in non-Western countries. In some, perinatal mood disorders are practically nonexistent. I had set up the abundant support I knew I would need. My husband is on leave. My parents and in-laws have visited. My brother has visited twice. We have a full-time caregiver, and our two older kids have begun preschool. Help abounds. And yet I still feel sad, ragged, and alone.

My therapist, Sarah, offers a metaphor—the common cold. You can read about what a cold is, how you catch it, and what it's like in your body, she says. You can talk to people about how it felt to be ill. You can learn all there is to know about colds. None of this is the same as getting sick.

When my baby is ten weeks old, I tell Sarah that I feel like I'm only just now beginning to attach to him. His smiling helps. He is beginning to cry less. He cried so much. Screamed, really. I talk about how I would go to him, enfold him into me for warmth and milk, often without making eye contact or speaking. Maybe he felt my discomfort, my stress and inner hollowness as I moved awkwardly, interacting with him robotically without eye contact or cooing love sounds.

Walking home, I realize that I have become a patient and that I need to be one. I stop at the store and emerge with a bag of roast chicken and prepared vegetables tucked underneath my arm. The muggy air now has a kick of chill. Did this just happen? I haven't really been outside. The Halloween decor goes up in shifts as peer pressure trickles down blocks. My neighbors' stoops are ensconced with arachnids. Halloween in Brooklyn is awesome but also scary if you're a small child unskilled at navigating the distinction between fantasy and reality. My middle son keeps asking if the spiders will get us, even as he also knows that they are pretend and won't. Ben texts a photo of the kids at a playdate. My heart shoots to my throat. They appear happy, if underdressed for the October chill, surrounding a table set for a tea party. The baby is strapped to Ben in a sling. On the street I pass gray-haired men with babies attached to them and watch smiling crowds part to let them through.

Sarah believes I'm experiencing feelings of aggression. When she says it, I picture something angry and physical and male—a football player, a movie villain. She assures me it's normal. I'm someone for whom that is and will continue to be important to hear. When Sarah says aggression, she doesn't mean violent or physical behavior, but rather the feeling of being fed up and resentful. Maybe these feelings prevented me from bonding with this baby as early as I did with the other kids, or maybe life is just busier now, more complicated. He fusses so much and at such a shrill pitch that I google "colic" for the first time. Does it last for three hours? I don't know. I'm not timing it. I'm living one never-ending day.

I resent that Ben is using his three-month paternity leave on home tasks. Repairs and organizing closets. Are to-do lists something he does to manage anxiety? Sarah asks me. I say yes but that I think they also create more of it. I realize that they are burnishing my own. There is also the research I'm steeped in, the articles about how, in hetero-sexual partnership, dads contribute far less at home than moms do. I'm primed for all the ways structural sexism creeps into our lives, which is ironic, as it doesn't creep into so much as frame them. I re-solve to show my work more—like it's a math problem. Copy Ben on school and scheduling emails. Deputize him to find Halloween cos-tumes. When he texts to ask the oven's potato-roasting temperature, reply with: Look it up?

I'm in a forest that I can't spot because I'm counting each twig.

It will be weeks before I learn that my insurance barely pays any-thing for therapy anyway.

THE MOMS IN MY SURVEY MENTIONED ANXIETY THREE TIMES AS often as depression. About sixty of them said anxiety was the hard-est part of pregnancy and childbirth. During pregnancy, they wor-ried for their babies' health. "I couldn't see inside!" one mom said. Some feared miscarriage or pregnancy loss after having experienced it before; others stressed because they were new to pregnancy and felt clueless. Many prayed for their babies' safety, far more often than they did for their own. Some feared the unknown: What would childbirth be like?

Another predominant cause of anxiety among my survey respon-dents was the disconnection between expectations and reality. "I didn't understand what was happening to my body," one woman said. "I had anxiety pretty bad." The unanticipated anxiety made mothers feel blindsided. They were unfamiliar with anxiety symptoms and didn't realize how common they are. Screening for the conditions was patchy at best. "Feeling out of control" was a common response from the anxious.

For some women, gender and race contributed to how others perceived their anxiety and how they felt it themselves. "They just thought I was a 'crazy new mom,'" said one woman, referring to hospital staff who cared for her. When asked how gender played a role in her birth story, another respondent said people think of "anxiety as a female trait." There was surprise that knowing postpartum anxiety could happen didn't prevent it from happening. "No amount of knowledge or preparation could yield it off," said my friend Alana. "It is chemical. It is hormonal. All of the self-knowledge I had could not fight off the wave of actual anxiety."

"I entered motherhood feeling like a failure who could not adequately support or nurture my children right out of the gate," said another mother.

Sarah, my therapist, tells me that poor sleep and dehydration can cause anxiety. I think she can tell I'm seeking an explanation.

BETWEEN 1939 AND 1962, BRITAIN LISTENED TO A BBC RADIO ADdress from Donald Winnicott, a psychologist who spoke plainly about mothers and children. The show tilled subjects like "jealousy" (normal, healthy, arising out of the fact that children love), "saying no" ("No because the stove is hot. No because I say so. No because I like that plant, implying that if the plant is pulled about, you won't love the baby so much for a few minutes"), and difficult feelings ("There are some people who are rather shocked if they find they can have other than loving feelings toward small children"). Winnicott was a titan in the midcentury British psychoanalytic movement whose ideas still feel new today. Psychologists and trainees remain fervent adherents of his theories and catchphrases, which appear in classrooms and treatment settings. Many connect with his realistic approach to motherhood.

"Do you, in fact, find it rather an irksome job, being a mother?" Winnicott asked Mrs. W on his radio program.

"Well, yes, I do, I think, on the whole, if I'm quite truthful," she replied.

Before migrating to psychology, Winnicott first worked as a pediatrician. He grew less interested in children's bodies ("assuming as one usually can do their physical health") than in their interior lives and the lives of their mothers. His talks, too, progressed from "infant feeding to infant mother mutual involvement." Yet, as he spoke through the radio, his identity remained secret, due to mandates—unimaginable in America—against doctors advertising. He inspired the far more famous pediatrician, Benjamin Spock, who wrote the forward to one of his books, which sold some fifty thousand copies between 1964 and 1968.

It's notable that women marshaled Winnicott's ideas and persona and ushered them to a mainstream audience. Janet Quigley and Isa Benzie produced his radio address, while his second wife and frequent collaborator, Clare, edited his books.

Do you know about the good enough mother? Sarah asks in session, in her office, a windowless room in another therapist's house. Though the simple moniker feels warm and familiar, I do not.

Not good *enough*, like barely passing or hardly capable. *Good* enough, meaning succeeding, doing your best. Emphasis on good. You can't give them everything they need, that's literally impossible, Sarah says of my kids, of anyone's kids. Even if you could, it would mess them up. I've seen patients with parents who gave them so much that it hinders, it paralyzes kids because they can't do anything for themselves, she says. You need to *not* meet their needs sometimes, because that's how they learn to do for themselves. Good enough.

Winnicott devised the good enough mother theory to describe how mothers transition from initial total devotion to a baby's needs to allowing a baby to experience small, tolerable amounts of frustration—crying for a few minutes without being soothed, for example—so the baby will one day separate from the mother and soothe themself. "In time the baby begins to need the mother to fail to adapt—this failure being also a graduated process that cannot be learned from books," Winnicott explains. This concept that imperfect motherhood is, in fact, perfect motherhood resonates with modern mothers and their therapists.

I burrow into Winnicott, taken with this framing and questing for more reading to help me understand and feel my own feelings, my mental state. I'm partial to his radio addresses, which are more conversational and ruminative than his journal articles. Here, mothers love their babies and embrace their duty to care, but also, upon discovering they have "become hostess to a new human being who has decided to take up lodging," utter things like "Damn you, you little bugger." It's like he can see me toting my kids down the preschool stairs on a Friday afternoon, anticipating the very long forty-eight hours ahead.

In the radio addresses I meet a lesser-known mother figure of Winnicott's imagining who is adjacent to the good enough mother but gets conflated and confused with her, even by psychologists. BBC producer Isa Benzie invited Winnicott to give a series of nine talks to mothers, and the two went for a walk to brainstorm about them in the summer of 1949. Benzie was after a fresh, Winnicottian catchphrase to hook the audience, but she didn't let on. "I told her that I had no interest whatsoever in trying to tell people what to do. To start with, I didn't know," Winnicott later wrote of the encounter. He wanted to converse with mothers "about the thing that they do well, and that they do well simply because each mother is devoted to the task in hand," which is raising babies. "Ordinarily this just happens." They had walked twenty yards when Benzie said, "Splendid! The ordinary devoted mother."

Winnicott argues that you can't teach early mothering; it's a natural act. However, you can impede it. Take breastfeeding: if there isn't a bodily problem, he posits, mother-infant pairs don't need instruction. Doctors and nurses forcibly positioning baby to breast at the bedside disrupts the pair figuring out a feeding rhythm on their own. "Unthinking people will often try to teach you how to do the things which you can *do* better than you can be *taught* to do them," he writes. When doctors and nurses impose choreography, force the act, and don't revere or believe in moms enough, their meddling leaves a residue of doubt. Winnicott describes the ordinary devoted mother as one who does what her dependents need without schooling from experts or books. Accordingly, we become the ordinary devoted mother when we are left alone.

I can't help but wonder what Winnicott would make of the internet many of us haunt—that of parenting journalism, moms groups, mom-fluencers, newsletters, and listservs. I imagine he'd advise us to tread carefully if not ignore them entirely.

The ordinary devoted mother benefits not just individual families but society at large. It's a fact that humans depend on the ordinary devotion and contributions of mothers. Winnicott takes it further, linking her commitment to the creation of our world. "If this contribution is accepted, it follows that every man or woman who is sane ... is in infinite debt to a woman," Winnicott writes. Accepting this debt, he continues, quells our fear. However, not everyone accepts this. When we don't, there are consequences. Namely, a fear of dependence that can manifest as a fear of women, Winnicott writes:

> If our society delays making full acknowledgement of this depen-
> dence, which is a historical fact in the initial stage of development of
> every individual, there must remain a block both to progress and to re-
> gression, a block that is based on fear. If there is no true recognition of
> the mother's part, then there must remain a vague fear of dependence.
> This fear will sometimes take the form of a fear of WOMAN [his caps]
> and at other times will take less easily recognized forms, always in-
> cluding fear of domination. Traced to its root in the history of each
> individual, this fear of WOMAN turns out to be a fear of recognizing
> the fact of dependence.

Put differently, rejecting the immensity and importance of ordinary motherly devotion—our childhood dependence on moms—costs our society dearly. This rejection may be responsible for all that is broken in our world, according to writer Maria Popova's interpretation of Winnicott. "Our failure to recognize that indebted dependence is responsible for some of the most fundamental fractures of society—from the obvious manifestations, ranging from interpersonal malignancies like misogyny to societal maladies like sexism, to the subtler and more systemic symptoms affecting everything from social norms to political regimes," she writes in a 2016 essay. I want to hear in this its reciprocal: that were society to revere and accept its dependence on mothers, we could end sexism, war, structural misogyny, dictatorship, hunger, poverty, anti-intellectualism, climate change, and more.

Those who repress their fear of domination by women feel compelled to dominate, Winnicott insists. You could argue that this creates the patriarchal hegemony that sublimates women. Winnicott knew that we aren't primed to accept ordinary motherly devotion when he asked, "Is not this contribution of the devoted mother unrecognized precisely because it is immense?" Surely our society's rejection of the immeasurable contributions of ordinary devoted mothers undergirds our internal conflict around becoming them. We both expect and direct ourselves to sacrifice for our infants, only for society to despise and fear us for it, then sublimate and strip us of power. We too have internalized this fear of ourselves. We have shuttered the possibility of power, this ordinary ability not only to meet the needs of our offspring but also to create them, to grow them, godlike, from our own flesh. We internalize early motherhood as a sentence we serve, not power at all but sacrifice.

Enabling the ordinary devoted mother of Winnicott's imagining is a better-known concept that he calls the *primary maternal preoccupation*. He likens the primary maternal occupation to a psychiatric condition or an illness that presents as a "heightened sensitivity" to what our infants require. Our feverish care for babies consumes us, erases our own needs, but then, as if lifted by wind, disappears. We forget it, or more likely, according to Winnicott, we repress it.

This idea seduced me because it held the promise of my innate capability to mother. It's soul warming to be told that you're naturally good at something, particularly something that feels impossible. It had been deliciously easy to get caught in the swirl of books, experts, data, and online tools—to believe in their promise of knowledge when I felt utterly bereft. But primary maternal preoccupation quieted that noise. It wasn't preparation that would orient me in motherhood but nature—my DNA, my psyche, my very marrow. I love the poetry and ease of a mothering that can't be learned, that's just in us. Like emotions. Like love.

But soon I began to wonder: What if the foray into motherhood is marked not by ease and obsession but by disease and confusion? What if, when we become mothers, we don't feel devoted or capable? What do we do with stress, feelings of loss, ambivalence? We suffer, struggle, and question. Maybe natural attentiveness is not known in our bones. Alongside my own natural ability crept paralyzing anxiety. There's paltry space in Winnicott's framework for the complexity and mixed feelings of mothers themselves.

"I just don't think he likes us," said Rebecca Palmer, who became a mom to Sam at twenty-five and started a colic podcast. "My perspective that as a mom I would instinctively know how to settle my own baby was so wrong." The 4th Trimester Project recommends that the healthcare system treat mom and baby as a dyad—a technical term for a mom-baby pair—rather than as individuals, emphasizing that they form a unit needing attention and care. "They aren't treated as dyads in the US currently," project researcher Kristin Tully told me. "That doesn't make sense." Tully gives the example of breastfeeding, which is bidirectional. Winnicott too insists that "ordinarily" after the baby's birth the mother and baby become one—"to a large extent she is the baby and the baby is her," making any separation or differing experience impossible. Good-bye, mixed feelings. The dyad frame recognizes that babies' and mothers' needs are inextricable. To me it also acknowledges, if sheepishly, that mothers are such a repudiated class that they must meld with their infants to receive any acknowledgment of their needs and experiences at all.

I KNEW NOTHING ABOUT BIRTH TRAUMA WHEN I USED THAT WORD to describe what I felt after my first childbirth. The speed and intensity floored me. I didn't have time to adjust to the idea of my daughter leaving my body, let alone the reality of it. Speeding to the hospital in an Uber, breathing unnaturally in the way my doula instructed, trying to intentionally suck her back in, rather than push her out, so she wouldn't be born on the car floor, felt new. We made it there and commandeered an elevator. I signed the consent form permitting the midwife to deliver my daughter after she was already lying on my chest, mouth pecking around for my nipple. Later, everyone said I was lucky that I didn't have to endure a long labor, which is true, I guess. But being told to feel lucky blots out the trauma of water breaking to infant shrieking in less time than it takes to watch a feature film, of narrowly missing having her in my bed, in a car, of being a person one minute and a mother the next.

As a nurse wheeled me to a recovery room, I tried to express what I was feeling. I was vibrating with sadness, hollowness. I had been ruptured. There had been a person living in my body, now there was not.

Do you have the baby blues? the nurse asked, worried.

I stammered, feeling threatened. I walked back my display of emotion.

Just surprised?

She said that if I was feeling depressed, I should tell somebody. I couldn't name what I was feeling. It was a slurry of sadness, elation, shock, fear. It took more than half an hour for my midwife to close what I later learned was a labial tear. She stitched me up while I examined this new daughter with sideburns, eyebrows, toenails. My joy and trauma were tangled. I didn't have postpartum depression, I had just given birth and become a mom.

Psychotherapist Peter Levine calls trauma "perhaps the most avoided, ignored, belittled, denied, misunderstood and untreated cause of human suffering." Childbirth is a trauma minefield. When you do it for the first time, you're more likely to experience trauma, according to Cheryl Beck, a nurse and academic who began studying birth trauma in 2000. Beck has studied and published on the topic more than anyone else I could find. She defines birth trauma as when a person is stripped of dignity or confronts an actual or threatened serious injury to themselves or their unborn child as birth unfolds. She has interviewed thousands of women who have experienced this, and they tell her it made them feel "betrayed," "terrified to the core of my being," and "abandoned and alone."

"If I had to use one image that women share with me to try and help me understand their traumatic birth, it's that they felt raped on the delivery table with everybody watching and no one offering to help," Beck told me. "I've heard that so many times."

When I first heard about traumatic birth, I assumed it was rare. But a third of women describe their birth experiences as traumatic. My survey found a slightly higher number—about 39 percent. Beck says birth trauma does not stem from the kind of birth you have but from your relationship to the experience. She gave me an example: Two women undergo emergency cesareans. One develops birth trauma or PTSD, while the other does not. What's the difference? "Birth is stripped of these systematic layers of caring," she says. "Women don't feel cared for during labor and delivery. They talk about being stripped of their dignity. They're not communicated with. Once a birth is over and if the baby's Apgars are good, it's considered a success by everybody's account. But no one wants to focus in on what the mother had to go through to give birth to that healthy baby. Women are systematically stripped of these protective layers while they're in labor." Trauma occurs when birthers' bodies and boundaries are violated, when they are left in the dark, and when it seems like nobody cares. It's akin to the other ways in which women are traumatized—harassment, assault, provocation, abuse.

When Winnicott expounded on good and ordinary mothers in the years after World War II, they were routinely traumatized during birth—rendered unconscious, cut open, violated. Later, they woke up and met their babies. Some were snookered into it. Others demanded the right to not suffer. My grandmother used to say, "I went to sleep, and I woke up a mom." I would laugh at this. It was delivered like a punchline.

Women didn't know that taking a baby from their body as they lay drugged and asleep could cause trauma and PTSD. Mothers have suffered for generations in ways we're only beginning to understand, but one thing is certain: their suffering is not past. It's also ours.

WHEN KRYSTA DANCY BEGAN PRACTICING THERAPY IN ROSEville, California, in 2005, she saw all kinds of patients. But after giving birth to her son, she began attracting new moms in earnest. In response to cultural mores that demand we transition to motherhood alone, many of us instead become magnets, pulling others toward us. Dancy began to notice peculiar symptoms during their treatment. They experienced flashbacks, nightmares, hyperarousal, and reclusion. They struggled to fall asleep, then couldn't get out of bed. They felt fear, helplessness, horror. Their own infants triggered them. Dancy found this reminiscent of what her combat veteran patients experienced. They too suffered from flashbacks, nightmares, hyperarousal, reclusion—textbook symptoms of post-traumatic stress disorder.

But Dancy's training told her the moms couldn't have that condition. Crucially, neither the mothers nor their infants had survived the conflict of war, a near-death experience, or serious injury, ineluctable criteria for PTSD that Dancy learned in school. Their deliveries were clinically uneventful.

"I was really confused," Dancy told me. "It looks like PTSD, and it talks like PTSD, and it feels like PTSD, but it's not supposed to be PTSD. So, what is it?" At first, she wouldn't treat new moms for a condition that they weren't supposed to have. Instead, she tried therapies for postpartum anxiety and depression, with some success, but "it didn't really feel like it was hitting what they needed," Dancy recalled. She asked mentors, colleagues, and experts what to do. She attended book signings of famous trauma therapists to badger them for advice.

"I would be that annoying student who would wait in a book-signing line and be like, 'I have this quick question about trauma after birth, and if you know anything about it, and if anybody's doing work about it?'" She would get a sideways look followed by "I have no idea what you're talking about" or "I don't know what's happening in the birth room, but I assume it's not good." This troubled Dancy. "It's important to say that most of them were older men," she recalled.

Men have long dominated the field of psychology and the American Psychiatric Association, which publishes the *Diagnostic and Statistical Manual (DSM)*, the mental health bible the field uses to identify and treat mental illness. Male researchers and therapists saw trauma in people who looked, talked, and acted like them—but not in women, who looked, talked, and acted differently and whose lives involved childbirth. In the twentieth century, men in professional organizations defined categories of trauma and what would become PTSD. Not only were labor and delivery outside their lived experience, they were also unseen and unknown by the culture at large. Recall that for much of the twentieth century many American women themselves weren't even awake and attendant for their own births. Just like the obstetrical dilemma—theorized and popularized by male evolutionary biologists and anthropologists who saw a flawed female pelvis but did not themselves give birth—trauma experts first legitimized PTSD from an entirely male vantage point.

The PTSD condition was born to describe suffering in a narrow, specific population of people: military veterans, mostly men. PTSD was officially added to the third edition of the *DSM* in 1980. The condition has been defined as occurring when a person has "experienced, witnessed, or [been] confronted with an event or events that involved actual or threatened death, serious injury, or a threat to the physical integrity of the self or others" and responded with "intense fear, helplessness or horror." But those who created the original PTSD diagnosis envisioned rare events as the cause: war, torture, rape, the Holocaust, the bombings of Hiroshima and Nagasaki, natural disasters (earthquakes), and human-caused disasters (car accidents).

Dancy realized that even though her patients who were moms didn't meet the official criteria, they were experiencing all the symptoms of PTSD. She began to treat them with the techniques she had successfully applied to veterans: therapies that allowed people to process events that get stuck on a loop. The moms got better. They referred others to her. "Trauma is the specialty that chose me," Dancy said.

The fifth edition of the *DSM* affirmed what Dancy already understood—that people didn't have to confront death for their trauma to count as PTSD. A woman could have PTSD after her baby was born, even if her birth seemed unremarkable. But what birth is unremarkable? What birth doesn't feel like what one imagines dying to be—holy, otherworldly, a transformation?

The definition of PTSD has since evolved to include experiencing or witnessing a traumatic event, or even just hearing of one. It wasn't until 2010, though, that researchers demonstrated, for the first time, in a large longitudinal study published in the journal *Psychological Medicine*, that childbirth caused PTSD. A 2012 study in the journal of the German Society of Gynecology and Obstetrics reaffirmed this finding. This research alerted psychologists to a new version of an old condition, one distinct to new moms.

We now know that PTSD is common—more than twice as common in women as in men. About 4 percent of men will get PTSD during their lifetimes, while 10 percent of women will. Yet experts believe these figures undercount, in part because mainstream narratives about PTSD still center men.

Flashbacks, nightmares, numbing detachment, reclusion, fear, and dread are PTSD symptoms that can manifest in anyone. Traumatic birth is the inciting event that can cause PTSD postpartum, also called P-PTSD. P-PTSD usually appears within a month of childbirth, however, clinicians see symptoms occurring beyond that time frame.

Some 9 percent of birthing people experience full-blown PTSD, according to the advocacy group Postpartum Support International. Mental health experts think these are conservative figures. Women either don't self-report or downplay what, to psychologists, are obvious markers. But birthing people aren't to blame. They're busy with new babies. They shouldn't have to diagnose themselves. Their healthcare providers are failing them.

"We're missing a lot of the women who really do have PTSD. A lot of women are not getting diagnosed with PTSD who really should be," said Tracey Vogel, an obstetric anesthesiologist who is also a trained counselor for rape and domestic violence survivors. Her colleagues at West Penn Hospital in Pittsburgh sometimes send her pregnant people with trauma histories so that she can help them as they prepare for birth. But this kind of arrangement is exceptionally rare.

Getting a P-PTSD diagnosis can be a Sisyphean task. Health professionals responsible for new mothers aren't looking for this. Many don't know how to treat postpartum patients. Too often, P-PTSD gets conflated or confused with other better-known mental health conditions. Providers might even make P-PTSD worse by treating the wrong problem.

Sharon Dekel, a professor of psychology at Harvard Medical School, told me about a mom in one of her studies who had given birth at a Massachusetts hospital. The hospital practiced rooming-in, a policy encouraging new moms to keep their infants in recovery with them overnight rather than sending them to a nursery, to facilitate bonding. The mom experienced birth trauma and refused to hold her baby. The nurse continued to insist. But Dekel told me that pressuring a mom to hold a baby whose very existence is a trauma trigger "is very, very dangerous for somebody who is already feeling so bad and might be on the verge of developing P-PTSD."

OBs, nurses, midwives, doulas, and pediatricians aren't trained to identify trauma. They don't look for it during prenatal visits, nor do they screen for it postpartum. They don't know that a trauma history makes birth trauma and P-PTSD more likely. They don't know what questions to ask. They might screen for postpartum depression, or, more likely, they'll assume that this time is hard for everyone and that stress will clear on its own.

In the 2010 study that first showed birth could cause PTSD, researchers controlled for preexisting PTSD, depression, and anxiety and concluded that "the findings indicate that PTSD can result from a traumatic birth experience." Two years later, researchers in Austria found a high incidence of PTSD in pregnant people who had given birth before, stating, "The potential consequences of PTSD diagnosed in pregnancy had never been investigated." They reported that the majority of their subjects—83 percent—had experienced at least one previous traumatic event in their lifetime. This finding suggests that pregnant people's trauma histories should be taken, and new parents should be screened for trauma and P-PTSD after birth, Vogel says. But our medical settings don't routinely record trauma histories. Hardly anyone screens women for PTSD after they give birth. Of the dozens of hospitals and OBGYN practices I spoke to in reporting for this book, not one said trauma screening was standard procedure. Sometimes someone with special training, like Vogel, is on a hospital's staff, and colleagues informally send them patients on the side. That's lucky and uncommon.

If a provider wants to diagnose the condition, she must give her patient one of the many existing PTSD screening tools. They are mostly checklists that assess the condition's symptoms. None are designed for new mothers. The PTSD checklist for the *DSM-5*, the edition published in 2013 that broadened the disorder to include non-life-threatening experiences, was developed by the National Center for PTSD of the US Department of Veterans Affairs. There is a military version and a civilian version. Neither targets the nuances of birth trauma.

Meanwhile, P-PTSD is commonly misdiagnosed as postpartum depression and anxiety. While the diseases are comorbid, they are distinct, says Dekel, whose lab studies how P-PTSD acts in the brain. "PTSD is a different condition than depression. It's different not only because there are different symptoms but because we know there are different biological changes that are part of the condition," she told me, like high cortisol levels and brain scan abnormalities.

This matters because when PTSD patients are treated as if they have *only* postpartum depression and anxiety, they don't improve, as Dancy found. For instance, in psychotherapy aimed to treat postpartum depression, a patient might be asked to relive her traumatizing birth. But for someone with P-PTSD, reliving the trauma might actually impede healing—it could retraumatize or simply be impossible. Instead, she might need a different kind of brain-based therapy to allow her to process the incident, like eye movement desensitization and reprocessing, or EMDR—which might not be available to her without a PTSD diagnosis.

Dekel says that while she's glad more moms are getting necessary depression diagnoses in recent years, PTSD sufferers are still being ignored. "We are kind of better able to detect women who might be at risk for depression, but nobody's actually, to my knowledge, identifying women who might be at risk for PTSD," Dekel said.

The hormonal, physical, and emotional changes mothers experience during the perinatal period are as unique in the human life cycle as they are frequently misunderstood. When we don't recognize and validate perinatal mental illness, birthing people suffer, but so do their families and society.

Postpartum depression's inclusion in the *DSM* and the advocacy, screening, and treatment that followed that designation could be a roadmap for P-PTSD awareness and diagnosis. Postpartum depression first arrived in the *DSM* as "major depressive disorder, with postpartum onset" in 1994. This update encouraged doctors to evaluate patients for a depression diagnosis within four weeks of birth. The most recent edition, *DSM-5*, lists "peripartum onset" as a category within a section on major depressive disorders, meaning pregnancy is included in the diagnostic period. Prior to this, many debated whether postpartum depression differed enough from depression in general to require its own entry, with specific diagnostic criteria. Some psychotherapists still don't believe that it does or that it warrants unique treatment.

The *DSM* entry isn't perfect. Despite its name, half of women eventually diagnosed with postpartum depression experienced symptoms during pregnancy. Postpartum Support International has lobbied to increase the diagnostic period to within six months postpartum, as symptoms can appear long after birth. That hasn't happened yet. But critically, the *DSM* inclusion legitimizes mental illness in pregnant people and new moms. There is more attention, diagnosis, and treatment because of it. It has also led to news coverage, societal awareness, research funding, and drug trials.

Dekel agrees that if postpartum-onset PTSD were included in the *DSM*, providers would be more likely to screen, diagnose, and treat new moms. She has published research on how P-PTSD threatens bonding between mom and baby, which can negatively impact a child's life in adulthood. "When bonding is impaired, that increases the risk of social-emotional problems, which are linked with mental health problems in adult offspring," Dekel said. She unspools the conflict to its natural, if cyclical, conclusion: the baby grows up and has a child of her own and passes the same difficulties down to her offspring, seeding "debilitating outcomes for our society." This is why including postpartum-onset PTSD could be so important—it could help break the cycle of intergenerational trauma the condition can cause.

Not everyone agrees with Dekel's assessment. When she began studying PTSD in postpartum people, her male colleagues, who were investigators in her research program, asked her, "Why do we need this PTSD with postpartum onset? Why is that important? Unless you tell me it's a different form of PTSD?" Dekel recalled. Her lab's research shows that, so far, P-PTSD *is* like PTSD. Military veterans and birthing people, as Dancy realized, present similar symptoms, which "concern intrusion about, and avoidance of, memories associated with the traumatic event."

Perhaps our society overlooks birth trauma and fails to diagnose P-PTSD because we can't fathom that childbirth could be unhappy, that a new mom could be sad or mentally ill. Or if it is imaginable, that it is unwelcome. Moms who describe birth as unsettling are blasted with social stigma. Postpartum women dodge censure by remaining silent. We're discouraged from expressing messy emotions when holding our fresh infants. We must dote unconditionally, coo and soften, shed anything too prickly or fierce. The single acceptable response to childbirth is the most joy you've ever known in your life.

MOST OF US ARE TOUSLED, ASKEW AFTER BIRTH, OUR ENTRY INTO
motherhood more untidy than serene. Negativity and sharpening
aren't welcome. But they should be. We are entitled to feel what we
feel and not what we're told to feel, especially by people who don't give
birth. A woman who shows negative emotions, walls herself off, or appears traumatized should not be quieted, judged, or ignored. Rocky
and tranquil starts are both valid.

This is why I appreciated feminist psychologist Joan Raphael-Leff's
2010 paper "Healthy Maternal Ambivalence." She gets this cultural
conundrum. And she assigns part of the blame to one of Winnicott's
ideas, the primary maternal preoccupation theory, in which postpartum moms naturally become focused almost exclusively on their babies. Raphael-Leff says that, although "some women do experience
primary maternal preoccupation," many do not, and by centering infants in this way Winnicott ignores the lived experience of flesh-and-
blood mothers.

Psychoanalysis "has long neglected maternal subjectivity," she
writes. To many male psychologists, Winnicott included, the mother
is merely an object on which infants project dependence. She is a
happy, servile being, seemingly without complexities or needs of her
own. This is the Madonna, the goddess, the ordinary devoted mother.
"So powerful was the psychoanalytic need to glorify motherhood,"
Raphael-Leff explains, "that the Madonna myth prevailed, seeing her
need to mother as symmetrical to the infant's need to be mothered."
Winnicott's primary maternal preoccupation theory "succumbed" to
this notion. Consequently, when we imagine successful motherhood,
it is this flawless face we see.

Winnicott described primary maternal preoccupation as unblemished, but also as an illness. Is illness required to mother well? We
know that hormonal shifts and brain changes quickly follow birth.
To me, it seems like one illness we suffer from as we transition to
motherhood could originate in the gap between the ordinary devoted mother—flattened into both her baby and a neglected care machine—and the normal, ambivalent, transitioning person.

We are still being crushed beneath primary maternal preoccupation's bulk. We are anxious, depressed, manic, withdrawn, traumatized, psychotic, obsessive, compulsive, persecuted. We are isolated from our families of origin or from communities we can rely on to lend support. We exchange ritual and care for screens. Those who are supposed to care for us, support us, give us courage, and even sometimes save our lives doubt that we are capable of birthing and mothering. We are inundated with headlines and experts. We look outside for so much. We can't look inside because we are too scared. We don't trust that space.

We know perfect motherhood is impossible, and yet we chase it. This effort requires a staggering cognitive dissonance to make it through each day. Any perceived failure to achieve perfection is unspeakable. Raphael-Leff cites a midcentury work of psychology research that described maternal anxiety, guilt, and self-blame as "natural female masochism." If the mother is not high performing and happy, she is deriving pleasure from her struggle and pain.

It shouldn't surprise us, then, that forbidding maternal ambivalence and subjective experience isn't benign. It compels us "to hide our conflictual and shameful negative feelings from professionals—and from ourselves," Raphael-Leff explains. This is where our distress lives. But we don't name it. Instead, we imbibe pedestaled Madonna depictions and feel shame.

Our maternal perfection quest may be global. In 2004, a qualitative study calling itself the first to investigate postpartum depression "across countries and cultures" illustrated the appeal and universality of denying maternal ambivalence. Researchers interviewed three distinct groups of people across eleven countries: mothers of five- to seven-month-old babies, the babies' fathers and grandmothers, and clinicians and health administrators. Focus groups convened at birth centers and hospitals in Austria, France, Ireland, Italy, Japan, Portugal, Sweden, Switzerland, Uganda, the United Kingdom, and the United States. The *British Journal of Psychiatry* published the results. Researchers found that loneliness, lack of emotional and social support, family and partner conflicts, tiredness, and struggles adapting to the work of baby care were common causes of unhappiness after delivery worldwide. What surprised researchers was that while "morbid unhappiness after childbirth comparable to postnatal depression is widely recognized," among the participants "no mention was made of negative feelings, of irritation or frustration." Study subjects universally suffered from distress but couldn't or didn't name it.

Primary maternal preoccupation, the Madonna myth, whatever you want to call it, thwarts us from accessing our natural, necessary ambivalence. We hide the feelings we have been socialized to feel are shameful, negative, and unflattering from those who love us, from professional question askers, and, most importantly, from ourselves.

Raphael-Leff pins such prevalent perinatal distress to factors "that conspire to prevent a woman from fulfilling her own maternal expectations." We chastise ourselves for not being better than we are. But, back to Winnicott, perhaps we are already good enough.

BEING A MOTHER "IS LIKE HAVING TO NAVIGATE ACROSS A FIELD covered with old car tires," claimed the writer Anne Lamott. In her essential recounting of the first year of her son's life, *Operating Instructions*, she describes the "worst night yet" when baby Sam won't stop crying for four hours. Even when the torturous wailing ends, it leaves a film over Lamott. She expresses how undermining this is, our ability to mother the being we made thwarted by their very programming: "The colic still makes me feel like a shitty mother, not to mention impotent and lost and nuts."

In 1967, after Winnicott's popular talks, psychologist Reva Rubin introduced the idea that maternal identity was "a complex cognitive and social process which is learned, reciprocal, and interactive." Maternal role attainment theory centers the mother and encourages postpartum care that does the same. Mothers learn to be mothers. They aren't born that way.

Childbirth instructor Mary Lynn Fiske-Dobell, who taught Ben and me the Bradley Method, described that feeling of wanting credit for motherhood, while being afraid that credit seeking was selfish or stole from the baby. "I remember people admiring baby. I was glad but also, 'Hey, wait a minute—do you realize what I just did?' Not only did I gestate this work of art, this magnum opus, then I gave birth to her, I'm making milk for her, I seem to know what to do," she said. "Can we admire me? No one does. It's complicated. Now, instead of being one, it's separate from you. You can feel lonely. And then you feel childish. Of course, the baby is great."

My heart palpitations eventually stopped. The baby slept more, and so did I. Amazing how tied these things were to my noticing baby greatness. Friends and interview subjects who launched early motherhood from a dark place were touchpoints. Talking to someone weekly helps. I still do it. The initial sting of suffering dulled, but sediment remains, that of having lived through something and come out of it.

CHAPTER 11
HOME BIRTH

IT TOOK A COUPLE OF SECONDS FOR ME TO MOVE FROM BEING asleep to being awake with the knowledge that my water had broken and I was in labor. There was a nascent sense of a clock ticking. A jumble of anticipation and fear. My heartbeat quickened. The last time my water had broken like this, before active labor started, I was at home, and it would be just two hours until I was in a hospital with a crying baby, my eldest, in my arms.

Ben didn't have to ask whether I was sure. He got up, kissed me, and texted Miriam, our midwife, who lives two blocks away. If you stand in the middle of our Brooklyn neighborhood and throw a rock, you'll almost certainly hit a home birth midwife. (But don't do that.)

Try to get some sleep, she texted back.

I felt a flash of hope that maybe labor wouldn't start for a few hours. I wanted her text to make that true. I hadn't been expecting a baby that night. I wasn't due until the following week. There were weekend plans. I had called incessantly to get a coveted dinner reservation for Ben's fortieth birthday and booked a sitter weeks ago. I planned to cook and freeze some meals and read the home birth picture book to my two older kids a few more times, just to make sure they were clear on what would go down. Good-bye to all of that.

It was shortly after midnight, a time I would never normally be awake. My other kids had been born during the day. I felt a twinge of regret that we would need to wake up our midwife, though waking up in the night to aid pregnant women in labor and deliver their children is her chosen profession. Babies come when they are ready. Clearly this one was fully baked. The good news about laboring overnight was that my daughter and my son, then ages four and two, were likely to sleep through it. One of my fears of birthing at home was being torn between trying to care for them and laboring, a time when I needed to care only for myself.

I lay on my side waiting. Ben got on the phone to alert our birth team. Unlike us, the room was ready, having been shorn of excess items and furnishings in preparation. It still contained our bed, dresser, and night tables, as well as a vintage "seed dispersal" poster that my father-in-law had nicked from the Swarthmore College library in 1973, its placement in the bedroom auspicious. We had moved a small couch and coffee table out of the room to allow for the birthing tub that we rented from Chaya, the go-to source for home birth pools in the area. We had to buy our own hose to fill it, because there's only so much sterilization she is willing to undertake when the rentals are returned. Understandable. The tub was still in a pile on the floor. It needed to be inflated and filled. Weeks earlier, Miriam had suggested we check our hot water to ensure we had enough to fill the tub.

Do you think we should blow up the tub? I asked, and by "we" I meant Ben.

Nah, we've got time, he said.

In my head I disagreed but didn't say so. Last time my water broke first, with no signs of labor prior, I had a precipitous birth that lasted barely over two hours. Ben knew this. He had been there. I decided to let it go. I knew that I had somewhere else to be, and that place was

not in this room but in my body. I needed sharp concentration to relax my limbs, to dive inward. But first, I would change my underwear
and the bedsheets. Everything was soaking wet. Ben placed the plastic
mattress cover over our bed, then topped it with a waterproof shower
curtain before sealing the bed with a sheet. No mattresses would be
destroyed in the arrival of this new life.

Unlike our home, hospitals are full of supplies designed for breaking skin and stopping blood. They know birth is accompanied by the
full range of human fluids. Thus, beds are swathed in sheets and what
amount to giant wee-wee pads. They have ice packs and heat packs
and peri bottles and Tucks pads and numbing cream and numbing
spray and just a coterie of numbing products, as well as diapers and
sanitary pads thick as sandwiches. We had to special order it all. Luck-
ily the prior week we had organized the items in bins and placed them
on our bedroom dresser, so they would be ready for the birth and after
the baby was born. In our room, which is often cluttered with our (and
our children's) things, the clean white bins, the negative space, the
deficit of junk—this visual soothed me in the days before labor began.

With the bed now prepared, I lay down again waiting for something
to happen. I remembered the feeling of contracting, my body being
wrung out like wet cloth by some unstoppable force, but it wasn't happening yet. Thinking about waiting caused a kick in my chest. I felt a
soft rumble. ... Could that have been a contraction? Maybe? I sipped
some water from a bottle by the bedside. I closed my eyes. Tried to
forget about the episode of *Succession* I had watched before bed. How
mean they all are! I dared to hope that a little more sleep was possible
but knew it wasn't. I pinched my eyes shut anyway.

I remembered the birth class adage: "You must learn to relax as if
your life depends on it." Because for however long you're laboring, it
kind of does. Our teacher strongly recommended that we support all
body parts with pillows so that when the contractions or rushes came,
we could experience them, supported, rather than grip our bodies and
fight them.

I thought about how, in that class, we pregnant women literally
practiced relaxing by lying on pillows, slacking taut bellies, untensing

rigid jaws, breathing deeply and rhythmically. I practiced this at home, too, back before I had any kids, and had the time to do something as luxurious as rehearse "letting go."

Now I returned to it instinctively. I lay sideways, propping body parts on different pillows, head and neck supported, bottom leg straight, top leg bent, cushions elevating my calf. There was no staring into a screen at the contraction timer app. That had been for knowing when to go to the hospital. This time, everyone was coming to us.

By the time our midwife and doula arrived, I was in the room and I wasn't. The contractions were coming now. The welling up, the wringing out. I breathed and moaned *Ahhh*. I had cried when I learned that that sound, the one that came naturally to me in labor, is also a name for God. Or so someone said on a podcast.

A strong contraction felt like a gale pouring through me, each muscle and organ squeezing on contact as if caught in an internal vise. I fought the tensing up in my muscles: pulsed calves, coiled toes, strained brow. I willed them to slack. I dropped into a liminal space, a loamy dark where all I could see were the stripes inside my eyelids, the round sound of my voice the only noise in the room. *Ahhh. Ahhh. Ahhh.*

Sounds like these are the music of birth. They are a physiologic necessity, moving the baby through the body. How often they were misunderstood in the hospital. My laboring sounds and movements appeared to be pain or panic. They invited doctors and nurses to intervene because they believed that something was wrong.

Miriam entered the room's periphery quietly with her midwife things. No booming voice announcing her presence, no orders or wires or tubes. Later, she listened to the baby's heart with a small Doppler device, earpieces the size of nickels. But mostly she watched me silently. She didn't touch me. She trusted me to do my thing.

THE PUSHING PHASE OF MY FIRST BIRTH FELT LIKE A FORCE. IT FELT automated. An untamable tide crashing through my being. Nobody coached me or counted. My body was overcome by a gripping urge and pushed on its own, and shortly after there was a baby. I hadn't realized that was a thing.

In labor, we talk about pushing a baby out without understanding the anatomy and physiology of that action. The uterus is the body's largest muscle group, and its strength is astounding. Imagine an oblong basket woven around a baby with a small opening at one end. The basket is the uterus, the opening is the cervix. The basket is strong, yet pliable. The cervix is shut for most of pregnancy, then it uncorks (sometimes slowly, other times all at once) to allow the baby out.

During active labor, the long muscles that run parallel along the length of the uterus contract and shorten, while the smaller, perpendicular muscles of the cervix relax and lengthen. In tandem these efforts eventually open, or dilate, the cervix. Imagine slowly pulling a turtleneck sweater over your head. Visualizing the movement of the uterine muscles during labor was important for me to allow the intense feeling of that action to happen, ideally with my aid, and if nothing else without my resistance.

When I was admitted to the hospital to have my second baby, the nurse told me that they would allow me to push once I had dilated to ten centimeters. I remember thinking, OK, but it seemed like a strange thing to say—that *they* would allow *me* to push. This instruction hadn't come up during prenatal appointments. The speed with which my first child was born offered no time for my body to be messed with. There was no waiting for permission. I had experienced what I would later learn is called the fetus ejection reflex. My daughter was born when my body decided, frankly, to shoot her out. Which is why, exactly two years later, I was miffed that the medical staff told me I could only push at their command. Still, I wanted to appease, so I was willing to try.

You can push now, said the obstetrician, once he had determined that I had reached the obligatory ten centimeters. A nurse directed me to the exam table with its back reclined halfway. I climbed onto it as she and a colleague watched. They encouraged me into a lithotomy position—supine on a table, legs spread and feet raised into stirrups, a posture that one midwifery professor dubbed "the stranded beetle." I didn't realize until later that my body hadn't selected that shape—they cajoled me there.

The doctor and nurses looked at the monitor, not at me, waiting for that quaking green line to build. One, two, three … push! someone instructed, before I knew what was happening. I tried. But the count caught me off guard. It felt so strange, being told to push, rather than my body pushing for me.

You can do better than that, a nurse said.

Directed pushing, also known as Valsalva pushing, with closed glottis breathing—or holding the breath at a contraction's outset and keeping it in while bearing down hard—is an inescapable part of hospital birth. It's also the effort we witness in nearly every mainstream interpretation of childbirth, featured in films like *Knocked Up, Father of the Bride, Juno,* and *What to Expect When You're Expecting.* In these depictions, sweat gushes, veins pop, docile femininity is tossed to the floor. The doctor seems like the only sane person in the room. "It feels like I'm shitting a knife!" screams Amy Poehler's character in *Baby Mama.* Valsalva pushing's traction in Hollywood mimics maternity wards, where the practice is ubiquitous.

Coached pushing's prevalence doesn't indicate its success. Medicine has had cause to doubt its universal application since at least the mid-twentieth century, when evidence against it began to emerge. A leading champion of spontaneous second-stage labor was Constance L. Beynon, who, in 1957, published a paper collecting evidence for it. "For many years now I have adopted the practice of allowing my patients to follow their own inclination in the second stage, forbidding all mention of pushing by those in attendance," she wrote. Beynon quotes a doctor who inadvertently witnessed a birth without coached pushing, calling into question the prototypical second stage of labor. The doctor had been stalling a first-time mother's labor so a colleague, the mother's doctor, could arrive. The doctor and nurses did this by "ignoring the patient's early straining efforts" and not coaching her to push. But when the baby's head reached the pelvic floor, it began to emerge on its own. "The baby was born with practically no effort on the part of the patient and an intact vagina and perineum. The peacefulness and obvious ease of the birth were most impressive," the doctor wrote in 1950.

Beynon had researched women with conditions that precluded them from pushing—physical disability, heart defects—and found that they frequently labored with ease. She tested the method in a clinical trial of one hundred women giving birth for the first time at Sussex Maternity Hospital in Brighton, a seaside town in England. Attendants were instructed to avoid coached pushing. Uttering the word *push* excluded cases from the study. The results were remarkable: eighty-three of the one hundred women allowed to push spontaneously birthed their babies that way, and in just one hour. "About 80 percent of laborers ... are able to deliver themselves instinctively with little more straining than is required in the process of defecation," Beynon observed in a paper sharing her clinical trial's results.

Beynon pleaded "for a more vigorous policy to eliminate hurry and unnecessary straining from the conduct of the normal second stage of labor" and recommended that "sound obstetric practice should aim primarily at giving every woman a reasonable chance to achieve complete normality." In her own deliveries, she continued, as she had been doing for many years, to forbid unnecessary pushing on command.

When her work was virtually ignored, she lambasted her colleagues, who "seem to consider it their function to aid and abet and even coerce the mother into forcing the fetus as fast as she can through her birth canal." Almost twenty-five years later, another landmark study found that spontaneous pushing improved the fetus's access to oxygen during labor's second stage. Some in the field hoped that medical professionals would pay more attention this time, as the findings of the new study—that a hands-off approach benefits babies—might have been more salient to hospitals than Beynon's discovery that it allowed easier labors for mothers. But the new work also failed to alter hospital management of the second stage of labor, which remains directed and controlled to this day.

I didn't know any of this lying in the extremely suboptimal lithotomy position in the delivery room. Motivated by criticism and the stares of hospital staff, the next time I had a contraction, I pushed. I felt a gush. The sack broke, amniotic fluid soaking the paper that crinkled beneath me. There was a pause. Then, before I knew what was happening, my whole body began to shake and seize. My back flung against the reclined exam table. Someone, probably a nurse, quickly shoved a supply cart out of the way. The footrest flew down with a clang, shortening the length of the table, to allow providers better access to the baby's head as it widened my perineum. My son flew out so fast that the doctor caught him with one hand, a first for each of us. The nurses who scrambled to get in place rolled their eyes. Later, I wanted to apologize for my body, its need to push that bypassed my consciousness, my control. Then later still I changed my mind.

I experienced the fetal ejection reflex in both my first and second births. It sounds mythical, but not only can it happen, it's common. I'm not an anomaly. The fetal ejection reflex can look like the birthing person is "on another planet" or that she goes from being in her body to holding a baby in seconds. Nevertheless, fetal ejection is often thwarted. Hurdles include, but are not limited to, vaginal exams, bright lights, noise, constant disturbances, fundal pressure, electronic monitoring equipment, eye contact, lack of privacy or trust, too much verbal communication (even reassurances and certainly coached pushing), and, tellingly, according to one midwife, Marianne Littlejohn, the "masculinization of the birth environment," meaning how men design and control the birth space as well as their sheer presence there.

Taken together, this list defines the American hospital birth experience. The disturbance of physiologic birth is the norm. We are told when to push rather than pushing when our bodies demand it. Maybe the fetal ejection reflex would be commonplace if birthing bodies weren't fucked with so much.

In the decades since Beynon's work was published, more evidence has affirmed spontaneous pushing's benefits. Allowing laboring people to push when they want helps them conserve energy during a process that demands more than they have ever expended in their lives. It shortens the amount of time spent actively bearing down, allowing for rest between parts of the labor process. More tests have confirmed improved oxygenation to the fetus and better Apgar scores at birth. Following the laboring person's own rhythms decreases operative deliveries and protects against episiotomy and tearing. It also just makes sense. Why would I, or anyone, push on command when my body doesn't want to, when I can push with great (and in my case near-total) assistance from my body when it does?

It isn't just that there are benefits to spontaneous pushing, or laboring down, as it's called. Directed pushing in a supine position can be harmful. It requires birthers to work against gravity, pushing the baby uphill. It increases the incidence of abnormal fetal heart rate, which can lead to interventions like cesarean or assisted deliveries with forceps or vacuum. Directed pushing in the lithotomy position can threaten perineal integrity because it closes the vaginal opening—according to one nurse, by up to 70 percent—and it can tire out a laboring person unnecessarily. Especially since, if she were to wait and rest, she would receive aid from gravity and her own urges.

This and other important perinatal research was formally collected in 1993 as the Cochrane Pregnancy and Childbirth database—an effort by evidence-based medicine boosters in the UK to put all the high-quality randomized clinical trials about birth in one place. They had hoped that improving access to research would engender evidence-based care. Shortly afterward, in 1994, the Association of Women's Health, Obstetric and Neonatal Nurses launched an effort at several hospitals intended to replace directed Valsalva pushing in the lithotomy position with laboring down. The evidence was there, but so was the gap in practice. Physicians were instructed to wait until laboring women felt the urge, or the head was visible, before asking them to push. They were forbidden from forcing anyone into a supine position. Supporting and honoring the natural pattern of labor's second stage was the goal.

Researchers found that doctors struggled to relinquish control and to dispense with counting to ten and commanding moms to push. The providers perceived the second stage as "too long" and hurried it. They didn't understand how to support spontaneous pushing, and they undermined their own nurses' attempts to offer that method of care. Use of the supine position endured. Most facilities failed.

It's unclear when and how directed pushing became the norm. One theory is that birth advocates in the midcentury developed Valsalva pushing to combat the difficulty of birthing in the routine supine position and used it to speed delivery and to preempt episiotomy and forceps births by giving physicians something else to do—count rather than cut.

"Given the history of the medicalization of childbirth, it is likely that intervening in the spontaneous process of labor and birth arose out of physicians' perceived need to manage and control a process they believed was inherently dangerous for both the mother and the baby," wrote Canadian midwife and nursing professor Kathryn Osborne.

Coached pushing isn't bad across the board. It can be a useful tool in some births. "Coached pushing works extremely well for some people and they are really grateful for the guidance and support," says doula and PhD Megan Davidson. "For other folks it is distracting, confusing, or feels counter to the cues they are getting from their body. Like everything about our experiences in childbirth, the issue is not whether coached pushing is a beneficial technique but rather the universal application of it," she explains.

Almost all the research comparing directed and spontaneous pushing promotes the latter. Notably, none of it reflects women's actual preferences—what they desire or reject in their own births. It's a familiar thread throughout birth research. Instead, studies focus on whether a particular type of pushing lengthens the second stage of labor. This tracks with a system in which quicker births mean more births, and more births mean more money.

Directed pushing in the supine position remains the status quo in hospitals across the country, despite the trove of evidence—academic and anecdotal—that disproves its usefulness and highlights its risks. Rather than integrating the best science, which also happens to put women in the driver's seat, hospitals that privilege directed pushing do so to maintain control.

There are providers who support laboring down and births led by women's bodies and urges. These births are most likely to occur in the 10 percent attended by midwives. And, of course, spontaneous

pushing in the nonlithotomy position is common practice when birthing at home.

WHEN I TELL HER I'M HAVING MY THIRD BABY AT HOME, MY NEIGH-
bor, an ER doctor, recommends that I talk to an obstetrician about it.

For permission? I ask, resistance welling up.

For information, she says.

You're right here if I need you, I joke.

We stand beneath the trees in front of our homes. Ours is a Japanese
pagoda. Hers is shielded by a gingko, branches clasping a plastic bag for
the last few weeks. I read that it is only the female variety of the tree that
stinks. I know I don't need a doctor's permission to birth at home. But I
tell her asking is a good idea, first to be agreeable, but then I believe it.

A few days later I call Dr. P, the obstetrician who caught my son
with one hand and sees patients in an office that I can walk to. I pass it
daily as I'm out retrieving kids from school. I can't tell whether I want
advice or approval. Maybe I just want someone to talk with about my
forthcoming birth. Someone who knows about my body and my previous births.

His office is brick, Tudor looking, shaded by trees. I'm sweating,
six months pregnant. My stomach is swollen, and my belly button has
turned inside out. My two-year-old informs me that "it's broken."

The front desk is confused—I'm pregnant, but this is my first visit?
Where have I been? I'm just here for a consultation, I say. I'm giving
birth at home. Still, they want my insurance. I produce a card. Then I
sit and wait, staring at a television screen that doesn't show television,
just advertisements, including one for labiaplasty. A nurse invites me
to test the protein in my urine. I explain that I'm just here to talk. Do
I want them to go ahead and take vitals? Height, weight, blood pressure? No, I'm good.

The next place I wait is a room that smells like alcohol wipes. I hear
nurses chattering in the hallway about weekend plans. Dr. P greets me,
but he doesn't look like the man I remember, the one I had pictured in
my head. I confuse him with a defense attorney I interviewed once. I

think it's interesting that I repeatedly confuse these men, that I imagine my former obstetrician as much taller (that's the lawyer!) than he is. He has a warm smile and little hair.

How's it going? he asks, like a friend. So, you're having a home birth? You look great.

He asks who my midwife is, and I tell him, but no familiarity registers. He asks whether she has good experience with home births, and I tell him yes, two decades. She's one of the longest-working home birth midwives in New York City. Are there a lot of people doing it? He asks. I tell him there are. That I was surprised by how many choices we had, just in our neighborhood. Ben and I had met with three different home birth midwifery practices. Two of them were partnerships of women. I realize that I may know more about home birth in Brooklyn than he does.

Dr. P tells me that with my history—my "proven pelvis" having given birth twice before, my young age (You're young, he says. I think thirty-six is young. I'm still in that camp), and my overall health (gleaned from looking at me across a desk), that I should be fine. It would likely go easily for me, and I won't need the stuff that hospitals offer. Of course, I know all this. But I feel seen as he says it. I feel relieved.

Haltingly, I realize, now that I have his permission, his confidence, and de facto blessing, that this was the reason I came. I didn't seek out the nurse midwife who delivered my daughter at the same hospital, whose office is also a short walk from my home. I called the male obstetrician. The doctor. I wanted *his* endorsement. As we continue to talk, I realize the other reason I confuse Dr. P with the lawyer. They are both warm and practiced in eye contact, but both also interrupt me nearly every time I open my mouth, a tic I'm at once attracted to and repulsed by, that makes me feel both comforted and small.

Dr. P doesn't know about home birth, but he does know about emergent birth, so I ask whether, in the case of an emergency—which I do not for a moment anticipate. I'm having this baby at home, I repeat—he would personally take care of me at the hospital. I guess I still wanted to know whether he could keep me safe if things went crooked.

His eyes crinkle. The face he makes for bad news.

I can't do that, he tells me. He and my midwife don't have a formal collaborative agreement together, and therefore he won't see her patients. I ask if there's a home birth midwife Dr. P has a collaborative agreement with. There isn't. If we're not physically in the homes, it's hard for us to know what's actually happening. Philosophically, it doesn't make sense for us to absorb all that liability without really having control of the situation, he tells me. The problem with home birth is there's no regulation. There's so many different homes.

I understand this, and I don't.

I ask about my greatest fear: a hospital transfer during my home birth. I don't believe this will happen, but since it seems to be among the worst things that could, I ask him my burning question. If I arrive at the hospital, will I be able to exercise informed consent and refusal? Will I retain power over my own body and mind? He says of course, informed consent is always the priority.

But then he contradicts himself.

The only problem is, the scenario I see you going to the hospital for, you yourself are not going to have that mindset anymore, he explains. You're going to be stressed out. You'll be so nervous that something bad is happening that you'll just go in and be like "Please take care of me." That's what ends up happening. He says the women he has witnessed transferring from a home birth to a hospital arrive scared. They're like, "Do whatever you want." If you go in, he tells me, you're not going to be in a state where you're asking for these things. You're going to be like, "Please make sure I'm OK." He's telling me that if I unexpectedly enter the hospital, I won't be able to exercise informed consent. I will relinquish control of my own body. Not because of the place or people but because of me.

I thank him for his advice, and he reassures me that I can call anytime, that I would still be considered his patient, even though my pregnancy is being cared for elsewhere. Good luck, he says, before walking out the door.

MY MOM WAS CHASTISED FOR REFUSING AN EPIDURAL AT THE Atlanta hospital where my brother was born. She described it as a place
that would come at you with a needle the second you said ouch. Once
he was out, nurses treated her like an exhibit, coming from other
floors and departments to spy the nutcase who had dared to deliver
without drugs. They thought it couldn't be done. But it could, and she
had, and when I became pregnant for the first time, I knew I wanted
to deliver the same way. I wanted to feel it, whatever *it* was, even
though I was terrified.

Sometimes the fetal ejection reflex occurs *because* of a stressor. The
baby has descended into the birth canal, and the safest thing for her
and for her mother is to exit ASAP. I have wondered if this is why my
babies flew out—because we were no longer in the dark and quiet; we
had entered the hospital sanctum and were now under duress.

I realize my speedy births in a hospital setting contradict the more
popular occurrence, which is stalled labor upon hospital entry. This
still puzzles me. Questing for answers about why I birth like this was
unfulfilling and only unearthed more questions. I wondered whether
my first baby had been in danger. Did she need to get out fast? The
woman who encapsulated my placenta sent me dozens of photos of
it—the largest placenta she had ever seen, she said—before she dried
and pulverized it, preparations for fashioning it into pills. First of all, it
was a marvel: glistening like the cap of an exotic mushroom, covered
in branching striations of plums and pinks. I stared at it on my screen
for days. My doula looked at the photos too. That was when she noticed that the thick umbilical cord that inserts into the placenta was
separated into three branches. It wasn't inserted centrally, as is typical. I had what's called a velamentous cord insertion.

Internet research after I left the hospital told me that this condition could have been dangerous, threatening the lifeline to the baby in
utero. When I asked the midwife at my six-week postpartum checkup
about it and why we hadn't known about the cord insertion sooner,
she said that such a thing was nearly impossible to pick up on a pregnancy scan. But even if they had, she wouldn't have been concerned.
It isn't a problem until it's a problem, she said. Could this be why my

birth was so quick? Probably not, she said. But we can't really know. Where I have landed is that bodies have intuitive knowledge that must be listened to in birth—by birthers first and then by everyone else.

The fetal ejection reflex isn't a new discovery. Perinatal psychologist, Northwestern University professor, and mother of four Niles Newton spent more than thirty years studying the relationship between childbirth and environment, beginning in the 1950s. She first observed and named the fetal ejection reflex in her instructive work on how a hostile place affects birth for mice. In her first study, she rotated full-term pregnant mice between their dark nesting boxes and clear bowls containing paper soaked in cat urine to discern whether the latter (unfamiliar, stressful) environment affected their births. Fewer mice delivered their babies in the habitat with the cat pee than in their homey crates. In another study, Newton calculated the lengths of mouse labors as one group was disturbed while another was left alone. The disturbed group labored up to 70 percent longer than the mice who weren't bothered. She conducted a third experiment in which one group of laboring mice bounced between two familiar environments, while another toggled between two hostile ones. Mice laboring in uncomfortable places took three to four hours longer to deliver their pups. The group with the familiar environments and no disturbances birthed more easily, and their young were more likely to survive. Newton concluded that hostile environments shut down the fetal ejection reflex by stopping the flow of catecholamines—the adrenaline and dopamine that assist in birth. "Anything that interrupts or distresses a female mouse in labor lengthens labor and lessens the likelihood of a normal outcome," distills one commentary about Newton's work.

We are not mice. We have a significantly more complex design and heightened brain function. However, we too require a safe, stress-free birth environment. It can invite the fetal ejection reflex, our bodies essentially autopiloting the pushing phase. However, as this book has established, most of us birth in an environment that is not only suboptimal but outright antagonistic.

Conventional wisdom maintains that home birth is inherently dangerous, while hospital birth is inherently safe. Both assumptions are false. People with normal pregnancies (read: most people) can safely birth at home if they choose to. Hospitals pose greater threats to birthers with normal pregnancies because they rarely ever support physiologic labor and usually thwart it with unnecessary interventions that cause trauma and complications. Remember, you're almost four times more likely to have a C-section if you birth in a hospital rather than at home.

There are situations when birthing at a hospital could be a better choice than birthing at home. First and foremost, when a person decides that's where she wants to birth. Simple as that. If she wants to birth in a hospital, she should. In the presence of certain health factors—such as severe preeclampsia, insulin-dependent diabetes, clotting disorders, chronic high blood pressure, or a history of preterm birth—birthing in a hospital is indeed safer. People with these conditions might need access to a blood transfusion, induction, surgery, and NICU care. They aren't forbidden from birthing where they choose, of course, but birth location, like care provider and plan, is an individual decision made with multiple considerations. Rare cases and high-risk situations are the reason miraculous interventions exist, so that they are accessible when they are needed most. But, as we know, technological intervention is wildly overused—and abused.

MIRIAM AND MY HUSBAND WHISPERED, AS THEY BEGAN TO FUMBLE with the tub. I said nothing, though it was getting to be too late to move. Cori, my doula, arrived as I was in the middle of a contraction. The only illumination in the room was a string of tiny white lights. My friend Gwen, a filmmaker and birth photographer, snaked them into the inflated birth tub, expecting me to be there. By the time the tub had been inflated and filled with water, getting into it was impossible. The contractions were too consuming. I couldn't move.

Cori and Miriam, doula and midwife, sat on the bed near me, just watching. Ben knelt beside me, his "Rock the Vote" T-shirt clinging to his chest. My back began to ache. I mentioned this to Cori, who asked if I might want to try the shower. Our drain was clogged, rendering it out of commission. A to-do list item we were going to use the weekend to address. Another bathroom seemed so far away, too distant to travel to in that moment. Everything inside told me to stay put. Cori found a heat pack and pressed it to my sacrum as Miriam watched. When a contraction came, I would use my voice to bring myself into it, to move with the feeling. I relaxed my muscles and imagined moving the baby forward with full-throated sound.

I remember a distinct break in the contractions that felt like I had awakened from a deep sleep. I came to consciousness, greeted Cori, thanked her for the heat, reached for my phone. My nails ticked on the glass, navigating to Spotify. That was the last moment I felt firmly rooted in the room before the contractions began to roll into each other with no reprieve.

The fetal ejection reflex took over. This time I wasn't threatened or bothered. The room was dark, quiet, and safe. I labored in the exact spot where I awoke that same night from broken water. In fact, I had barely moved from that mattress divot. An inner intelligence told me not to. After rippling contractions, I felt like I was on another planet. Miriam witnessed the increasing intensity in my movements, the sounds I was making, and the strain in my face. She moved closer. She didn't speak. I felt Gwen's presence but didn't notice her or her camera.

I was overcome with the urge to push—as if my body was being puppeteered. The baby didn't come out in one motion like the other two had. It was like he got stuck. I felt that burning sensation, which I had previously heard called the ring of fire. It zapped me of strength and presence, and it sowed real doubt.

Ben dutifully grabbed the handheld mirror we had bought as part of our DIY birth kit. Look! he said. But I couldn't. I had wanted to theoretically, to see my baby emerge and catch the warm body in its earthly descent into my hands. But that was impossible. That was reality. I was somewhere else. Doubt, even thoughts of death, are a common indicator that the end of the active phase of labor is near. Humans are the unique mammals who need birth assistance. Our animal relatives all do it alone. But we need supporters, partners. Ideally those who recognize the signpost of doubt and help us navigate through it.

Reach down and feel the head, Miriam offered. It's the only thing she said to me that I remember. It felt warm, damp, soft. Pulsing with life. That charge launched me through the doubt. Moments later there he was.

About a year before my son was born, I wrote a magazine feature about birth photography censorship on Instagram and Facebook. The social media companies classified images and videos of childbirth as pornography, deleting them from their platforms and reprimanding or removing those who post them. Some of those posters had built communities of followers in the tens and hundreds of thousands, gathering into their orbit people who wanted to witness what childbirth looks like, often for the first time. The online birth community lobbied to get the rules changed, created petitions, rallied supporters. The companies acquiesced, sort of. They still remove these profiles because sometimes humans police the sites, sometimes bots.

Getting lost in Birthstagram, I was struck by how moving birth images could be and how, for most of us, such images are the first or only births we witness before we ourselves give birth. They're educational tools and works of art. They involve nudity, so naturally they would be misunderstood and prohibited by structures whose relationship to the body is sheerly consumptive. I had grown increasingly jealous of people who posted their birth photos because my own births hadn't been captured in that way. I knew I wanted that this time. I wanted to see it later, as an outsider would. It's hard to savor the moment when you're doing it. Even discussing birth as something to want to do, rather than something that must be withstood, a means to an end, a necessary evil we are programmed to forget so we will repeat it, is to breach a cultural norm. Keeping the proof is radical. In my bed at home, my son arrived, and my friend Gwen snapped photos. They are some of the most precious ones I have.

She got images of baby crowning, sure. But she also captured what can be a very difficult shot to get. It's called a "half-in, half-out" in birth photography parlance. I'm centered in the image, mid-writhe, back arched and chin(s) flattened like a stack of pancakes. Because I'm screaming like I'm trying to crack glass. You can see my widened nostrils, the lens of my husband's glasses, and the arm and profile of Miriam, trying to catch my baby as he turns, his hair swishing. The next photo in the series is of Ben, me, and our baby, slick with vernix and blood. My eyes are closed and I'm smiling. Ben's hand cups our baby's matted hair. He's smiling and crying and pressing his forehead to the side of mine. I had bought a tasteful, forest-colored bralette to wear for the birth and in the photos, but it never made it out of the drawer.

The most power I've ever felt was during birth. Birthing at home, I didn't have to play defense. I didn't have to fight for the agency and permission to do it the way I wanted. That was everything. I now understand how birth can become an addiction, how some people end up with more kids than toes.

When I think about this now, when I hear that a friend or loved one is pregnant, I am overcome with want. First, I pray that the coercion, manipulation, and needless suffering won't touch them. Then, I wish for them support and the gift of being left alone to do the work of labor, to experience its magic and power. I want this for everyone.

ACKNOWLEDGMENTS

THIS BOOK IS A CAPSULE OF MY EPISODIC OBSESSIONS DURING AND after my pregnancies and childbirths. It's also a massive undertaking, and there are many to thank for its existence.

I'll start with the folks at Seal Press and Hachette who brought this book into being. Thank you, Emma Berry, Stephanie Blumenkrantz, Jessica Breen, Meghan Brophy, Katie Carruthers-Busser, Brian Distelberg, Lara Heimert, Emi Ikkanda, Jen Kelland, Chin-Yee Lai, Madeline Lee, Laura Mazer, Rachel Molland, Alcimary Pena, Kathy Steckfus, and Liz Wetzel. Thank you to my agents, Richard Pine and Eliza Rothstein. Thank you to Lisa Rubin and Tonya Pavlenko and their team at the New School, who analyzed my survey data with formidable expertise but also brought curiosity and care to the process.

Important conversations with countless people over the last decade informed this work—experts, luminaries, writers, confidantes, friends, neighbors, strangers. They include Aza Nedhari and the incredible team at MamaToto Village, Aviva Romm, Kavita Patel, Cori Pleune, Rachel Miller, Andrew Friedman, Jenny Reiner, Becky Friedman, Anne Juceam, Jenna Wallace, Molly Dickens, Corynne Cirilli, Holly Dunsworth, Rebecca Feldman, Sara Reardon, Tommy Rosen, Valeria Macías, Neel Shah, Holly Grigg Spall, Jessica Zucker, Eliza

Reynolds, Jennifer Weiss-Wolf, Dara Kass, Jane Van Dis, Jason Shen, William Frey, Malika Whitley, Kifah Shah, Heather O'Neil, Michele Filgate, Reshma Saujani, Elisabeth Sherman, and many others.

I joke that through writing this book, I have become a birth story whisperer. Even if we've just met, you will tell me your birth story within minutes. I believe that it is sacred to know birth stories and our duty to ask about others' births. My deep gratitude goes to the people who took my survey as well as to those who spent even more time sharing the intimate details of their births with me and answering my many questions. Alana Ain, Jenna Angst, Paige Cohen, Vanessa Coke Cohen, Sabrina Sikora Dommenge, Tamara Humphrey, LaToya Jordan, Lisbeth Kaiser, Ash Klaiber, Gwen Schroeder, Madhureeta Goel Southworth, and Shamia McGlip-Gallivan, thank you.

Thank you, Cyndi Stivers and Katrina Conanan, for supporting the seedlings of this book in the TED residency, and thank you to my residency classmates, who challenged me to clarify and expand my vision on this topic. Thank you to the International Women's Media Foundation for supporting my early reporting. Thank you to the Brooklyn Writers Space and the John Jermain Public Library in Sag Harbor for housing me while I worked.

Thank you to the Gaudets and the Yarrows for your encouragement. Thank you, Ruby, Oscar, and Dean for giving me these experiences to obsess about and ruminate on and for continuing to teach me and inspire my growth. Thank you, Rachel Chrystie, Arlene Fender, and Maria Lopez, for taking care of these small people I adore so that I can write.

Thank you, Ben, for catching our kids when they were born and for holding me, always.

NOTES

INTRODUCTION

Backes, Emily P., and Susan C. Scrimshaw, eds. *Birth Settings in America: Outcomes, Quality, Access, and Choice*. National Academies Press, 2020.

Beck, Cheryl. "Middle Range Theory of Traumatic Childbirth: The Ever-Widening Ripple Effect." Global Qualitative Nursing Research. March 2015.

Block, Jennifer. *Pushed: The Painful Truth About Childbirth and Modern Maternity Care*. Da Capo Press, 2007.

Febos, Melissa. *Body Work: The Radical Power of Personal Narrative*. Catapult Press, 2022.

Gaskin, Ina May. *Ina May's Guide to Childbirth*. Bantam Books, 2003.

Gregory, Elizabeth C. W., Michelle J. K. Osterman, and Claudia Valenzuela. "Changes in Home Births by Race and Hispanic Origin and State of Residence of Mother: United States, 2018–2019 and 2019–2020." National Vital Statistics Reports. Centers for Disease Control and Prevention. December 2021. https://pubmed.ncbi.nlm.nih.gov/34895406.

Kitzinger, Sheila. *A Passion for Birth: My Life: Anthropology, Family, and Feminism*. Pinter & Martin Ltd., 2015.

Lukpat, Alyssa. "These Mothers Were Exhausted, So They Met on a Field to Scream." *New York Times*. January 23, 2022. www.nytimes.com/2022/01/23/us/mom-scream-massachusetts-pandemic.html.

MacDorman, Marian F., Eugene Declerq, Howard Cabral, and Christine Morton. "Is the United States Maternal Mortality Rate Increasing? Disentangling Trends from Measurement Issues." *Obstetrics & Gynecology* 128, no. 3 (September 2016): 447–455.

Olgin, Alex. "Male OB-GYNs Are Rare, but Is That a Problem?" *Morning Edition*. NPR. April 12, 2018. www.npr.org/sections/health-shots/2018/04/12/596396698/male-ob-gyns-are-rare-but-is-that-a-problem.

Perrine, Cria G., Katelyn V. Chiang, Erica H. Anstey, Daurice A. Grossniklaus, Ellen O. Boundy, Erin K. Sauber-Schatz, Jennifer M. Nelson. "Implementation of Hospital Practices Supportive of Breastfeeding in the Context of COVID-19 United States, July 15–August 20, 2020." *Morbidity and Mortality Weekly Report.* November 27, 2020. www.cdc.gov/mmwr/volumes/69/wr/mm6947a3.htm.

Rich, Adrienne. *Of Woman Born: Motherhood as Experience and Institution.* W. W. Norton & Company, 1986.

Sgaier, Sema, and Jordan Downey. "What We See in the Shameful Trends on U.S. Maternal Health." *New York Times.* November 17, 2021. www.nytimes.com/interactive /2021/11/17/opinion/maternal-pregnancy-health.html.

Yarrow, Allison. "The Mother Load Survey." 2019.

Chapter 1. Welcome to Pregnancy

Baskett, T. F., and F. Naegele. "Naegele's Rule: A Reappraisal." *British Journal of Obstetrics and Gynaecology* 107, no. 11 (November 2000): 1433–1435.

Baskett, Thomas. *Eponyms and Names in Obstetrics and Gynecology.* Cambridge University Press, 2019.

Briden, Laura. *Period Repair Manual: Natural Treatment for Better Hormones and Better Periods.* CreateSpace, 2015.

Caughey, Aaron B., Vandana Sundaram, Anjali J. Kaimal, Yvonne W. Cheng, Allison Gienger, Sarah E. Little, and Jason F. Lee. "Maternal and Neonatal Outcomes of Elective Induction of Labor." *Agency for Healthcare Research and Quality Evidence Reports/Technology Assessments* 176 (2009):1–257.

Committee on Obstetric Practice, American College of Obstetricians and Gynecologists. "Methods for Estimating the Due Date." Committee Opinion No. 700. *Obstetrics & Gynecology* 129 (May 2017): e150–154. www.acog.org/clinical/clinical-guidance/committee -opinion/articles/2017/05/methods-for-estimating-the-due-date.

"Contraceptive Use by Method, 2019." Department of Economic and Social Affairs. United Nations. www.un.org/development/desa/pd/sites/www.un.org.development.desa.pd/ files/files/documents/2020/Jan/un_2019_contraceptiveusebymethod_databooklet.pdf.

Declercq, Eugene R., Carol Sakala, Maureen P. Corry, Sandra Applebaum, and Ariel Herrlich. *Listening to Mothers III: Pregnancy and Birth.* Childbirth Connection, May 2013. www.nationalpartnership.org/our-work/resources/health-care/maternity/listening-to -mothers-iii-pregnancy-and-birth-2013.pdf.

Dekker, Rebecca, and Anne Bertone. "The Evidence On: Due Dates." Evidence Based Birth. Last updated November 24, 2019. https://evidencebasedbirth.com/ evidence-on-due-dates.

Dekker, Rebecca, and Anne Bertone. "Evidence On: Inducing for Due Dates." Evidence Based Birth. Last updated February 24, 2020. https://evidencebasedbirth.com/ evidence-on-inducing-labor-for-going-past-your-due-date.

Dimont, Ethel. *The Hidden Injury: One Woman's Life-Changing Journey After a Brain Injury.* LuLu Press, 2011.

Dusenbery, Maya. *Doing Harm: The Truth About How Bad Medicine and Lazy Science Leave Women Dismissed, Misdiagnosed, and Sick.* Harper One, 2018.

Gantz, Sarah. "Coronavirus Is Changing Childbirth in the Philadelphia Region, Including Boosting Scheduled Inductions." *Philadelphia Inquirer.* August 12, 2020. www .inquirer.com/health/coronavirus/coronavirus-childbirth-scheduled-inductions-phila delphia-hospitals-pregnancy-pandemic-20200812.html.

Gardosi, Jason, Tracey Vanner, and Andy Francis. "Gestational Age and Induction of Labour for Prolonged Pregnancy." *British Journal of Obstetrics and Gynaecology.* August 19, 2005. https://doi.org/10.1111/j.1471-0528.1997.tb12022.x.

Grigg Spall, Holly. *Sweetening the Pill: Or, How We Got Hooked on Hormonal Birth Control.* Zero Books, 2013.

Hendrickson-Jack, Lisa. *The Fifth Vital Sign: Master Your Cycles and Optimize Your Fertility.* Fertility Friday Publishing, 2019.

Jukic, Anne Marie, Donna D. Bair, Clarice R. Weinberg, D. R. McConnaughey, and Allen J. Wilcox. "Length of Human Pregnancy and Contributors to Its Natural Variation." *Human Reproduction* 28, no. 10 (October 2013): 2848–2855.

Karkowsky, Chavi. *High Risk: Stories of Pregnancy, Birth, and the Unexpected.* Liveright, 2020.

Khambalia, Amina Z., Christine L. Roberts, Martin Nguyen, Charles N. Albert, Michael C. Nicholl, and Jonathan Morris. "Predicting Date of Birth and Examining the Best Time to Date a Pregnancy." *International Journal of Gynecology and Obstetrics* 123, no. 2 (2013): 105–109.

Kiefer, Amy. "Your Due Date Is Wrong—So When Is Labor Most Likely?" *Expecting Science.* September 29, 2014. https://expectingscience.com/2014/09/29/your-due -date-is-wrong-so-when-is-labor-really-most-likely.

Mittendorf, Robert, Michelle A. Williams, Catherine S. Berkey, and Paul F. Cotter. "The Length of Uncomplicated Human Gestation." *Obstetrics & Gynecology* 75, no. 6 (June 1990): 929–932.

Morken, Nils-Halvdan, Kari Klungsøyr, and Rolv Skjaerven. "Perinatal Mortality by Gestational Week and Size at Birth in Singleton Pregnancies At and Beyond Term: A Nationwide Population-Based Cohort Study." *BCM Pregnancy and Childbirth* 14, no. 172 (May 2014). doi: 10.1186/1471-2393-14-172.

Smith, Gordon C. S. "Use of Time to Event Analysis to Estimate the Normal Duration of Human Pregnancy." *Human Reproduction* 16, no. 7 (July 2001): 1497–1500.

Wegienka, Ganesa, and Donna Day Baird. "A Comparison of Recalled Date of Last Menstrual Period with Prospectively Recorded Dates." *Journal of Women's Health* 14, no. 3 (April 2005): 248–252.

Yarrow, Allison. "The Mother Load Survey." 2019.

CHAPTER 2. FEAR OF DEATH

Block, Jennifer. *Pushed: The Painful Truth About Childbirth and Modern Maternity Care.* Da Capo Press, 2007.

Charles Smith, Margaret. *Listen to Me Good: The Life Story of an Alabama Midwife.* Ohio State University Press, 1996.

DeLee, Joseph. "The Prophylactic Forceps Operation." *American Journal of Obstetrics and Gynecology1*, no. 1 (October 1920): 34–44. www.sciencedirect.com/science/article /abs/pii/S0002937820900674.

DeLee, Joseph. "Symposium: To What Extent Should Delivery Be Hastened or Assisted by Operative Interference?" *American Journal of Obstetrics and Gynecology* 2, no. 3 (1921): 297–307.

Ehrenreich, Barbara, and Deirdre English. *For Her Own Good: Two Centuries of the Experts' Advice to Women.* Rev. ed. Anchor, 2005.

Ehrenreich, Barbara, and Deirdre English. *Witches, Midwives, and Nurses: A History of Women Healers.* Feminist Press, 1993.

"Global Progress and Projections for Maternal Mortality." Goalkeepers Report: The Future of Progress. Bill & Melinda Gates Foundation. 2022. www.gatesfoundation.org /goalkeepers/report/2022-report/progress-indicators/maternal-mortality.

"Preventing Pregnancy-Related Deaths." Centers for Disease Control and Prevention. April 13, 2022. www.cdc.gov/reproductivehealth/maternal-mortality/preventing -pregnancy-related-deaths.html.

Rich, Adrienne. *Of Woman Born: Motherhood as Experience and Institution.* W. W. Norton & Company, 1986.

Webb-Hehn, Katherine. "Midwifery Makes a Comeback in Alabama." *Scalawag.* September 3, 2018. https://scalawagmagazine.org/2018/09/alabama-homebirth-reproductive-justice.

Wertz, Richard W., and Dorothy C. Wertz. *Lying-in: A History of Childbirth in America.* Exp. ed. Yale University Press, 1989.

White House Conference on Child Health and Protection. Century Company, 1933.

Wolf, Jacqueline. *Deliver Me from Pain: Anesthesia and Birth in America.* Johns Hopkins University Press, 2009.

CHAPTER 3. FEAR OF PAIN

Bridges, Khiara. *Reproducing Race: An Ethnography of Pregnancy as a Site of Radicalization.* University of California Press, 2011.

Clark, Rebecca R. S., Nicole Warren, Kenneth M. Shermock, Nancy Perrin, Eileen Lake, and Phyllis W. Sharps. "The Role of Oxytocin in Primary Cesarean Birth Among Low-Risk Women." *Journal of Midwifery & Women's Health.* September 15, 2020. https://online library.wiley.com/doi/10.1111/jmwh.13157.

Daly, Deirdre, Karin C. S. Minne, Alweina Blignaut, Ellen Blix, Anne Britt Vika Nilsen, Anna Dencker, Katrien Beeckman, et al. "How Much Synthetic Oxytocin Is Infused During Labour? A Review and Analysis of Regimens Used in 12 Countries." *PLOS One* 15, no. 7 (July 28, 2020): e0227941.

Dick-Read, Grantly. *Childbirth Without Fear.* Heinemann Medical Books, 1949.

Epstein, Abby, dir. *The Business of Being Born.* Produced by Ricki Lake, Abby Epstein, Paulo Netto, and Amy Slotnick. New Line, 2008.

Gaskin, Ina May. *Ina May's Guide to Childbirth.* Bantam Books, 2003.

Hoberman, John. "The Primitive Pelvis: The Role of Racial Folklore in Obstetrics and Gynecology During the Twentieth Century." In *Body Parts: British Explorations in Corporeality,* edited by Christopher E. Forth and Ivan Crozier. Lexington Books, 2005.

Kaul, Bupesh, Manuel C. Vallejo, Sivam Ramanathan, Gordon Mandell, Amy L. Phelps, and Ashi R. Daftary. "Induction of Labor with Oxytocin Increases Cesarean Section Rate as Compared with Oxytocin for Augmentation of Spontaneous Labor in Nulliparous

Parturients Controlled for Lumbar Epidural Analgesia." *Journal of Clinical Anesthesia* 16, no. 6 (September 2004): 411–414.

King, Lily. *Writers and Lovers.* Grove Atlantic, 2020.

Makvandi, S., K. Mirzaiinajmabadi, N. Tehranian, H. Esmily, and M. Mirteimoori. "The Effect of Normal Physiologic Childbirth on Labor Pain Relief: An Interventional Study in Mother-Friendly Hospitals." *Maedica* 13, no. 4 (December 2018): 286–293.

McCutcheon, Susan. *Natural Childbirth the Bradley Way.* Plume, 1996.

Moura, Kathleen McCaul. "If Mother's Happy." *Granta.* September 10, 2017. https://granta .com/if-mothers-happy.

"Placebo." *Radiolab.* WNYC Studios. May 18, 2007.

Rich, Adrienne. *Of Woman Born: Motherhood as Experience and Institution.* W. W. Norton & Company, 1986.

Ryan, C. Anthony, Desmond MacHale, and Yvonne Cohen. "A Letter from George Boole and Victorian Attitudes Toward Pregnancy, Childbirth, and Breastfeeding." *Hektoen International: A Journal of Medical Humanities.* January 27, 2017. https://hekint.org /2017/01/27/a-letter-from-george-boole-and-victorian-attitudes-towards-pregnancy -childbirth-and-breastfeeding.

Teysko, Heather. "Pregnancy and Childbirth in Tudor England." Englandcast.com. May 22, 2017.

CHAPTER 4. CHILDBEARING HIPS

Betti, Lia, and Andrea Manica. "Human Variation in the Shape of the Birth Canal Is Significant and Geographically Structured." *Proceedings of the Royal Society B* 285, no. 1889 (October 24, 2018): 20181807.

Declercq, Eugene R., Carol Sakala, Maureen P. Corry, Sandra Applebaum, and Ariel Herrlich. *Listening to Mothers III: Pregnancy and Birth.* Childbirth Connection, May 2013. www.nationalpartnership.org/our-work/resources/health-care/maternity/listening -to-mothers-iii-pregnancy-and-birth-2013.pdf.

Dekker, Rebecca. "Evidence On: Suspected Big Babies." Evidence Based Birth. January 2018. https://evidencebasedbirth.com/wp-content/uploads/2018/01/Big-Babies -Handout.pdf.

Dunsworth, Holly M. "There Is No 'Obstetrical Dilemma': Toward a Braver Medicine with Fewer Childbirth Interventions." *Perspectives in Biology and Medicine* 61, no. 2 (September 5, 2018): 249–263.

Dunsworth, Holly M., Anna G. Warrener, Terrence Deacon, and Herman Pontzer. "Metabolic Hypothesis for Human Altriciality." *Proceedings of the National Academy of Sciences* 109, no. 38 (August 29, 2012): 15212–15216.

Hoberman, John. "The Primitive Pelvis: The Role of Racial Folklore in Obstetrics and Gynecology During the Twentieth Century." In *Body Parts: British Explorations in Corporeality,* edited by Christopher E. Forth and Ivan Crozier. Lexington Books, 2005.

Karp, Harvey. *The Happiest Baby on the Block: The New Way to Calm Crying and Help Your Baby Sleep Longer.* Bantam, 2003.

Margalit, Ruth. "How Harvey Karp Turned Baby Sleep into Big Business." *New York Times Magazine*. April 18, 2018. www.nytimes.com/2018/04/18/magazine/harvey-karp-baby-mogul.html.

Margulies, Megan. "Should Pregnant Women Be Induced at 39 Weeks?" *Washington Post*. June 27, 2016. www.washingtonpost.com/national/health-science/should-pregnant-women-be-induced-at-39-weeks/2016/06/27/e1bb9d16-27fe-11e6-b989-4e5479715b54_story.html.

McCoubrey, Carmel. "Alice Stewart, 95; Linked X-Rays to Diseases." *New York Times*. July 4, 2002. www.nytimes.com/2002/07/04/world/alice-stewart-95-linked-x-rays-to-diseases.html.

Pavličev, Mihaela, Roberto Romero, and Phillip Mitteroecker. "Evolution of the Human Pelvis and Obstructed Labor: New Explanations of an Old Obstetrical Dilemma." *American Journal of Obstetrics and Gynecology* 222, no. 1 (January 2020): 3–16.

Rosenberg, Karen, and Wenda Trevathan. "Birth, Obstetrics, and Human Evolution." *British Journal of Obstetrics and Gynaecology* 109, no. 11 (November 2002): 1199–1206.

Warrener, Anna G., Kristi L. Lewton, Herman Pontzner, and Daniel E. Lieberman. "A Wider Pelvis Does Not Increase Locomotor Cost in Humans, with Implications for the Evolution of Childbirth." *PLOS One* 10, no. 3 (March 11, 2015): e0118903.

Yin, Steph. "Why Textbooks May Need to Update What They Say About Birth Canals." *New York Times*. October 27, 2018. www.nytimes.com/2018/10/27/health/birth-canals-evolution.html.

Chapter 5. It's Better to Be Cut

Albers, Leah, Kay D. Sedler, Edward J. Bedrick, Dusty Teaf, and Patricia Peralta. "Midwifery Care Measures in the Second Stage of Labor and Reduction of Genital Tract Trauma at Birth: A Randomized Trial." *Journal of Midwifery & Women's Health* 50, no. 5 (September–October 2005): 365–372.

Amorim, M. M., Isabela Cristina Coutinho, Inês Melo, and Leila Katz. "Selective Episiotomy vs. Implementation of a Non-episiotomy Protocol: A Randomized Clinical Trial." *Reproductive Health* 14, no. 1 (April 24, 2017): 55.

Begley, C., K. Guilliland, L. Dixon, M. Reilly, C. Keegan, C. McCann, and V. Smith. "A Qualitative Exploration of Techniques Used by Expert Midwives to Preserve the Perineum Intact." *Women Birth* 32, no. 1 (February 2019): 87–97.

Declercq, Eugene R., Carol Sakala, Maureen P. Corry, Sandra Applebaum, and Ariel Herrlich. *Listening to Mothers III: Pregnancy and Birth*. Childbirth Connection, May 2013. www.nationalpartnership.org/our-work/resources/health-care/maternity/listening-to-mothers-iii-pregnancy-and-birth-2013.pdf.

Dekker, Rebecca. "The Evidence On: Birthing Positions." Evidence Based Birth. Last updated July 11, 2022. https://evidencebasedbirth.com/evidence-birthing-positions.

Dekker, Rebecca. "The Evidence on the Top 5 Ways to Prevent Tearing During Childbirth." Evidence Based Birth. Fall 2021. https://evidencebasedbirth.com/replay-of-the-evidence-on-the-top-5-ways-to-prevent-tearing-during-childbirth.

Dekker, Rebecca. "Top 5 Ways to Prevent Tearing During Childbirth." Evidence Based Birth. October 2021. https://evidencebasedbirth.com/wp-content/uploads/2021/10/Protecting-the-Perineum-Handout.pdf.

Deliktas, Ayse, and Kamile Kukulu. "A Meta-analysis of the Effect on Maternal Health of Upright Positions During the Second Stage of Labour, Without Routine Epidural Analgesia." *Journal of Advanced Nursing* 74, no. 2 (February 2017): 263–278.

Huang, Jing, Yu Zang, Li-Hua Ren, Feng-Juan Li, and Hong Lu. "A Review and Comparison of Common Maternal Positions During the Second-Stage of Labor." *International Journal of Nursing Sciences* 6, no. 4 (March 2019): 460–467.

Johnson, Kimberly Ann. *The Fourth Trimester: A Postpartum Guide to Healing Your Body, Balancing Your Emotions, and Restoring Your Vitality.* Shambhala, 2017.

Klein, Michael C., Robert J. Gauthier, Sally H. Jorgensen, James M. Robbins, Janusz Kaczorowski, Barbara Johnson, and Marjolaine Corriveau. "Does Episiotomy Prevent Perineal Trauma and Pelvic Floor Relaxation?" *Online Journal of Clinical Trials* (July 1, 1992): Doc. 10.

Kopas, Mary Lou. "A Review of Evidence-Based Practices for Management of the Second Stage of Labor." *Journal of Midwifery & Women's Health* 59, no. 3 (2014): 264–276.

McCutcheon, Susan. *Natural Childbirth the Bradley Way.* Plume, 1996.

Mizrachi, Yossi, Sophia Leytes, Michal Levy, Zvia Hiaev, Shimon Ginath, Jacob Bar, and Michal Kovo. "Does Midwife Experience Affect the Rate of Severe Perineal Tears?" *Birth Issues in Perinatal Care* 44, no. 2 (2017): 161–166.

Thacker, Stephen B., and David H. Banta. "Benefits and Risks of Episiotomy: An Interpretative Review of the English Language Literature, 1860–1980." *Obstetrical Gynecological Survey* 38, no. 6 (June 1983): 322–338.

Ugwu, Emmanuel Onyebuchi, Eric Sunday Iferikigwe, Samuel Nnamdi Obi, George Uchenna Eleje, and Benjamin Chukwuma Ozumba. "Effectiveness of Antenatal Perineal Massage in Reducing Perineal Trauma and Post-partum Morbidities: A Randomized Controlled Trial." *Journal of Obstetrics and Gynaecology Research* 44, no. 7 (2018): 1252–1258.

Wertz, Richard W., and Dorothy C. Wertz. *Lying-in: A History of Childbirth in America.* Exp. ed. Yale University Press, 1989.

Willyard, Cassandra. "Episiotomy Rates Are Dropping, but Some Doctors Still Snip." *New York Times.* April 30, 2019. www.nytimes.com/2020/04/17/parenting/episiotomy.html.

CHAPTER 6. SURGICAL STRIKE

Some reporting for this chapter appeared in an opinion piece I wrote for the *New York Times* titled "One Hospital's Plan to Reduce C-sections: Communicate," June 5, 2019, www.nytimes.com/2019/06/05/opinion/hospital-cesarean-section.html.

Aggarwal, Reena, Avery Plough, Natalie Henrich, Grace Galvin, Amber Rucker, Chris Barnes, William Berry, Toni Golen, and Neel T. Shah. "The Design of 'TeamBirth': A Care Process to Improve Communication and Teamwork During Labor." *Birth: Issues in Perinatal Care* 48, no. 4 (December 2021): 534–540.

Alfirevic, Z., D. Devane, G. M. Gyte, and A. Cuthbert. "Continuous Cardiotocography as a Form of Electronic Fetal Monitoring for Fetal Assessment During Labour." Cochrane Database of Systemic Reviews. February 3, 2017.

American College of Obstetricians and Gynecologists and the Society for Maternal-Fetal Medicine. "Obstetric Care Consensus: Placenta Accreta Spectrum." *Obstetrics & Gynecology* 132, no. 6 (December 2018): e259–e275.

Baranauskas, Carla. "Dr. Orvan W. Hess, 96, Dies; Developed Fetal Heart Monitor." *New York Times*. September 16, 2002. www.nytimes.com/2002/09/16/us/dr-orvan-w-hess-96-dies-developed-fetal-heart-monitor.html.

"Birth by Design: Are Celebs Too Posh to Push?" Fox News. January 13, 2015. www.foxnews.com/story/birth-by-design-are-celebs-too-posh-to-push.

Brietbart, Andrew, and Mark Ebner. *Hollywood, Interrupted: The Case Against Celebrity*. John Wiley and Sons, 2004.

Cassidy, Tina. *Birth: The Surprising History of How We Are Born*. Grove Press, 2007.

Cheyney, Melissa, Marit Bovbjerg, Courtney Everson, Wendy Gordon, Darcy Hannibal, and Saraswathi Vedam. "Outcomes of Care for 16,924 Planned Home Births in the United States: The Midwives Alliance of North America Statistics Project, 2004 to 2009." *Journal of Midwifery & Women's Health* 59, no. 1 (2014): 17–27.

Clark, Steven, Jonathan B. Perlin, Sarah Fraker, Jamee Bush, Janet A. Meyers, Donna R. Frye, and Thomas L. Garthwaite. "Association of Obstetric Intervention with Temporal Patterns of Childbirth." *Obstetrics and Gynecology* 124, no. 5 (2014): 873–880.

Cohen, Wayne, and Emanuel A. Friedman. "Guidelines for Labor Assessment: Failure to Progress?" *American Journal of Obstetrics and Gynecology* 222, no. 4 (2020): P342.E1–342.E4.

Declercq, Eugene R., Carol Sakala, Maureen P. Corry, Sandra Applebaum, and Ariel Herrlich. *Listening to Mothers III: Pregnancy and Birth*. Childbirth Connection, May 2013. www.nationalpartnership.org/our-work/resources/health-care/maternity/listening-to-mothers-iii-pregnancy-and-birth-2013.pdf.

Dekker, Rebecca. "The Evidence on Fetal Monitoring" Evidence Based Birth. Updated March 21, 2018.

Dekker, Rebecca, and Anna Bertone. "The Evidence on: Fetal Monitoring." Evidence Based Birth. July 17, 2012. https://evidencebasedbirth.com/fetal-monitoring.

"Fetal Monitoring Market Worth $5.2 Billion by 2026—Exclusive Report by MarketsandMarkets." PRNewswire. March 31, 2021. www.prnewswire.com/news-releases/fetal-monitoring-market-worth-5-2-billion-by-2026--exclusive-report-by-marketsandmarkets-301259353.html.

Fields, Amanda, and Rachel Moritz. *My Caesarean: Twenty-One Mothers on the C-section Experience and After*. The Experiment, 2019.

Friedman, Emanuel. "Primigravid Labor: A Graphicostatistical Analysis." *Obstetrics & Gynecology* 6, no. 6 (1955): 567–589.

Hamesmäki, Erja. "Vaginal Term Breech Delivery—A Time for Reappraisal?" *Acta Obstetricia et Gynecologica Scandinavica* 80, no. 1 (March 2001): 187–190.

Hannah, Mary E., Sheila A. Hewson, Ellen D. Hoddnett, Saroj Saigal, and Andrew R. Willan; Term Breech Collaborative. "Planned Caesarean Section Versus Planned Vaginal

Birth for Breech Presentation at Term: A Randomised Multicentre Trial." *Lancet* 356, no. 9239 (October 21, 2000): 1375–1383.

Horsager-Boehrer, Robyn. "Why a Scheduled C-section After 35 Might Be Too Risky." *Medblog*. UT Southwestern Medical Center. April 23, 2019. https://utswmed.org/medblog/cesarean-over-35-risks.

Korb, Diane, François Goffinet, Aurélien Seco, and Catherine Deneux-Tharaux; EPI-MOMS Study Group. "Risk of Severe Maternal Morbidity Associated with Cesarean Delivery and the Role of Maternal Age: A Population-Based Propensity Score Analysis." *Canadian Medical Association Journal* 191, no. 13 (April 1, 2019): E352–E360.

Kotaska, Andrew. "Inappropriate Use of Randomized Trials to Evaluate Complex Phenomena: Case Study of Vaginal Breech Delivery." *British Medical Journal* 329, no. 7473 (October 30, 2004): 1039–1042.

Long, Tony. "Jan. 14, 1794: First Successful Cesarean in U.S." *Wired*. January 14, 2011. www.wired.com/2011/01/0114caesarean-first-us.

Martin, Joyce A., Brady E. Hamilton, Michelle J. K. Osterman, and Anne K. Driscoll. "Births: Final Data for 2019." *National Vital Statistics Reports* 70, no. 2 (March 23, 2021): 1–51.

Matthews, Anna Wilde, Tom McGinty, and Melanie Evans. "How Much Does a C-section Cost? At One Hospital, Anywhere from $6,241 to $60,584." *Wall Street Journal*. February 11, 2021. www.wsj.com/articles/how-much-does-a-c-section-cost-at-one-hospital-anywhere-from-6-241-to-60-584-11613051137.

"MindChild Medical, Inc., Announces Results of National Fetal Monitoring Market Survey." BusinessWire. June 11, 2012. www.businesswire.com/news/home/20120611005095/en/MindChild-Medical-Inc.-Announces-Results-of-National-Fetal-Monitoring-Market-Survey.

Neal, Jeremy L., Nancy K. Lowe, Karen L. Ahijevych, Thelma E. Patrick, Lori A. Cabbage, and Elizabeth J. Corwin. "'Active Labor' Duration and Dilation Rates Among Low-Risk, Nulliparous Women with Spontaneous Labor Onset: A Systematic Review." *Journal of Midwifery & Women's Health* 55, no. 4 (July–August 2010): 308–318.

Placek, P. J., and S. M. Taffel. "Trends in Cesarean Section Rates for the United States, 1970–78." *Public Health Reports* 95, no. 6 (November–December 1980): 540–548.

Praderio, Caroline. "People Are Furious at Kate Hudson for Calling a C-section the 'Laziest' Thing She's Ever Done." *Insider*. September 13, 2017. www.insider.com/kate-hudson-said-c-section-is-lazy-2017-9.

Roosmalen, Jos van, and Tarek Meguid. "The Dilemma of Vaginal Breech Delivery Worldwide." *Lancet* 383, no. 9932 (May 31, 2014): P1863–1864.

Rutherford, Julienne N., et al. "Reintegrating Modern Birth Practice Within Ancient Birth Process: What High Cesarean Rates Ignore About Physiologic Birth." *American Journal of Human Biology* 31, no. 2 (February 10, 2019): 1–11.

Sartwelle, T. P., J. C. Johnston, and B. Arda. "A Half Century of Electronic Fetal Monitoring and Bioethics: Silence Speaks Louder Than Words." *Maternal Health, Neonatology and Perinatology* 3, no. 21 (November 21, 2017). doi: 10.1186/s40748-017-0060-2.

Seelbach-Goebel, B. "Twin Birth Considering the Current Results of the 'Twin Birth Study.'" *Geburtshilfe und Frauenheilkunde* 74, no. 9 (September 2014): 838–844.

Shute, Nancy. "Doctors Urge Patience, and Longer Labor, to Reduce C-sections." NPR. February 20, 2014. www.npr.org/sections/health-shots/2014/02/20/280199498/doctors-urge-patience-and-longer-labor-to-reduce-c-sections.

Smith, J., F. Plaat, and N. M. Fisk. "The Natural Caesarean: A Woman-Centered Technique." *British Journal of Obstetrics and Gynaecology* 115, no. 8 (July 2008): 1037–1042.

Weaver, Jane, and Julia Magill-Cuerden. "'Too Posh to Push': The Rise and Rise of a Catchphrase." *Birth* 40, no. 4 (December 2013): 264–271.

Whyte, Hilary, Mary Hannah, and Saroj Saigal; Term Breech Trial Collaborative Group. "Outcomes of Children at 2 Years of Age in the Term Breech Trial." *American Journal of Obstetrics and Gynecology* 189, no. 6 (December 1, 2003): S57.

Zhang, Jun, James Troendle, Umma M. Reddy, S. Katherine Laughon, D. Ware Branch, Ronald Burkman, Helaine J. Landy, et al. "Contemporary Cesarean Delivery Practice in the United States." *American Journal of Obstetrics and Gynecology* 203, no. 4 (2010): 326.e1–326.e10.

CHAPTER 7. CONSENTING YOU

For hospital episiotomy data, see "A Tale of Two Births in CA," California Maternal Quality Care Collaborative, www.cmqcc.org/qi-initiatives/supporting-vaginal-birth/tale-two-births-ca; and "Episiotomies," Leapfrog Ratings, https://ratings.leapfroggroup.org/measure/hospital/episiotomies.

Aciman, André. "Are You Listening? Conversations with My Deaf Mother." *New Yorker*. March 10, 2014. www.newyorker.com/magazine/2014/03/17/are-you-listening.

"Ancient Roman Surgical Instruments." Historical Collections at the Claude Moore Health Sciences Library. University of Virginia. 2007. http://exhibits.hsl.virginia.edu/romansurgical.

Committee on Gynecologic Practice. "The Utility of and Indications for Routine Pelvic Examination." Number 754. American College of Obstetricians and Gynecologists. October 2018. www.acog.org/clinical/clinical-guidance/committee-opinion/articles/2018/10/the-utility-of-and-indications-for-routine-pelvic-examination.

Dekker, Rebecca. "Evidence on Prenatal Checks at the End of Pregnancy." Evidence Based Birth. February 1, 2017. https://evidencebasedbirth.com/evidence-prenatal-checks.

Febos, Melissa. *Body Work: The Radical Power of Personal Narrative.* Catapult Press, 2022.

Lenihan, J. P., Jr. "Relationship of Antepartum Pelvic Examinations to Premature Rupture of Membranes." *Obstetrics & Gynecology* 63, no. 1 (1984): 33–37.

McDuffie, R. S., G. E. Nelson, C. L. Osborn, C. D. Parke, S. M. Crawmer, M. Orleans, and A. D. Haverkamp. "Effect of Routine Weekly Cervical Examinations at Term on Premature Rupture of the Membranes: A Randomized Controlled Trial." *Obstetrics & Gynecology* 79, no. 2 (1992): 219–222.

Tillman, Stephanie. "Consent in Pelvic Care." *Journal of Midwifery & Women's Health* 65, no. 6 (2020): 749–758.

"Trauma-Informed Care and Consent with Feminist Midwife, Stephanie Tillman." Podcast 180. Evidence Based Birth. June 9, 2021. https://evidencebasedbirth.com/trauma-informed-care-and-consent-with-feminist-midwife-stephanie-tillman.

Chapter 8. Mummy Tummy

Some reporting in this chapter appeared in articles I wrote for *Vox*: "What No One Tells New Moms About What Childbirth Can Do to Their Bodies," updated May 4, 2018, www.vox.com/science-and-health/2017/6/26/15872734/postnatal-care-america; and "The Post-Pregnancy Belly Problem That Nobody Tells Women About," updated May 12, 2018, www.vox.com/science-and-health/2017/12/22/16772580/diastasis-recti-pregnancy-mommy-pooch.

Bø, Kari, Bary Berghmans, Siv Mørkved, Marijke Van Kampen, eds. *Evidence-Based Physical Therapy for the Pelvic Floor: Bridging Science and Clinical Practice.* Churchill Livingstone/Elsevier, 2015.

Bowman, Katie. *Diastasis Recti: The Whole-Body Solution to Abdominal Weakness and Separation.* Propriometrics Press, 2017.

Doucleff, Michaeleen. "Flattening the 'Mummy Tummy' with 1 Exercise, 10 Minutes a Day." *Morning Edition.* NPR. August 7, 2017. www.npr.org/sections/health-shots/2017/08/07/541204499/flattening-the-mummy-tummy-with-1-exercise-10-minutes-a-day.

Doucleff, Michaeleen. "Getting to the Core of Exercises Said to Strengthen 'Mum Tum.'" NPR. August 20, 2017. www.npr.org/sections/healthshots/2017/08/20/542424977/getting-to-the-core-of-exercises-said-to-strengthen-mum-tum.

"50 Years of Physiotherapy." International Continence Society. February 20, 2020. www.ics.org/news/1047.

Hoffman, Jonathan, and Phillip C. Gabel. "The Origins of Western Mind-Body Exercise Methods." *Physical Therapy Review* 20, nos. 5–6 (2015): 315–324.

Igualada-Martinex, Paula. "ICS Updates on Continence Care: What's Hot in Physiotherapy After 80 Years." *Urology News* 20, no 3 (March/April 2016). www.urologynews.uk.com/features/features/post/ics-updates-on-continence-care-whats-hot-in-physiotherapy-after-80-years.

Nygaard, Ingrid, Matthew D. Barber, Kathryn Burgio, Kimberley Kenton, Susan Meikle, Joseph Schafer, Cathie Spino, et al. "Prevalence of Symptomatic Pelvic Floor Disorders in US Women." *Journal of the American Medical Association* 300, no. 11 (September 17, 2008): 1311–1316.

Pattee, Emma. "Are Kegels All We've Got?" *The Cut.* March 6, 2020. www.thecut.com/2020/03/are-kegels-all-weve-got.html.

"Pelvic Floor Disorders Affect Almost a Quarter of U.S. Women." National Institutes of Health. September 29, 2008. www.nih.gov/news-events/nih-research-matters/pelvic-floor-disorders-affect-almost-quarter-us-women.

Perrine, Cria G., Katelyn V. Chiang, Erica H. Anstey, Daurice A. Grossniklaus, Ellen O. Boundy, Erin K. Sauber-Schatz, and Jennifer M. Nelson. "Implementation of Hospital Practices Supportive of Breastfeeding in the Context of COVID-19—United States, July 15–August 20, 2020." *Morbidity and Mortality Weekly Report.* November 27, 2020. www.cdc.gov/mmwr/volumes/69/wr/mm6947a3.htm.

Price, Natalie, Rehana Dawood, and Simon R. Jackson. "Pelvic Floor Exercises for Urinary Incontinence: A Systematic Literature Review." *Maturitas* 67, no. 4 (2010): 309–315.

Sperstad, Jorun Bakken, Merete Kolberg Tennfjord, Gunvor Hilde, Marie Ellström-Engh, and Kari Bø. "Diastasis Recti Abdominis During Pregnancy and 12 Months After Childbirth: Prevalence, Risk Factors and Report of Lumbopelvic Pain." *British Journal of Sports Medicine* 50, no. 17 (2016): 1092–1096.

Spitznagle, Theresa M., Fah Che Leong, and Linda R Van Dillen. "Prevalence of Diastasis Recti Abdominis in a Urogynecological Patient Population." *International Urogynecology Journal* 8, no. 3 (March 2007): 321–328.

Stein, Amy. *Heal Pelvic Pain.* McGraw-Hill, 2009.

Stewart, Monica. "Obituary: Dorothy Mandelstam." *Independent.* February 5, 1997. www.independent.co.uk/news/people/obituary-dorothy-mandelstam-1277005.html.

Tibaek, Sigrid, and Christian Dehlendorff. "Pelvic Floor Muscle Function in Women with Pelvic Floor Dysfunction: A Retrospective Chart Review, 1992–2008." *International Urogynecology Journal* 25, no. 5 (May 2014): 663–669.

Vopni, Kim. *Your Pelvic Floor: A Practical Guide to Solving Your Most Intimate Problems.* Watkins, 2021.

Chapter 9. Breast Is Best

Some reporting in this chapter first appeared in my articles "Why Do We Understand So Little About Breastfeeding?" *Washington Post*, February 21, 2018, www.washingtonpost.com/news/posteverything/wp/2018/02/21/why-do-we-understand-so-little-about-breastfeeding; and "Support for Breastfeeding Moms Is Already Abysmal. The Pandemic Is Making It Worse," *USA Today*, October 1, 2021. www.usatoday.com/story/opinion/voices/2021/10/01/breastfeeding-covid-hospitals-support/5891176001.

Allers, Kimberly. *The Big Letdown: How Medicine, Big Business, and Feminism Undermine Breastfeeding.* St. Martin's Press, 2017.

Bobel, Chris. "Bounded Liberation: A Focused Study of La Leche League International." *Gender & Society* 15, no. 1 (February 2001): 130–151.

Cole, Ellen. *Breasts: The Women's Perspective on an American Obsession.* Routledge, 1998.

"Current Partners." American Academy of Pediatrics. www.aap.org/en/philanthropy/corporate-and-organizational-partners/current-partners.

D'Argenio Waller, Jessica. "There's a Racial Gap in Breastfeeding. Here's What You Need to Know." *Motherly.* August 20, 2021. www.mother.ly/black-lives-matter/racial-gap-breastfeeding.

Dockterman, Eliana. "COVID-19 Is Making New Moms Feel Even More Pressure to Breastfeed." *Time.* September 22, 2021. https://time.com/6098463/breastfeeding-covid-19-antibodies.

Feldman-Winter, Lori B., Richard J. Schanler, Karen G. O'Connor, and Ruth A. Lawrence. "Pediatricians and the Promotion and Support of Breastfeeding." *Archives of Pediatrics & Adolescent Medicine* 162, no. 12 (2008): 1142–1149.

Grayson, Jennifer. *Unlatched: The Evolution of Breastfeeding and the Making of a Controversy.* HarperCollins, 2016.

Hinde, Katie. "What We Don't Know About Mother's Milk." TED.com. March 28, 2017. www.ted.com/talks/katie_hinde_what_we_don_t_know_about_mother_s_milk.

Lerner, Sharon. "The Real War on Families: Why the U.S. Needs Paid Leave Now." *In These Times*. August 18, 2015. https://inthesetimes.com/article/the-real-war-on-families.

Martucci, Jessica L. *Back to the Breast: Natural Motherhood and Breastfeeding in America.* University of Chicago Press, 2015.

McKinney, Chelsea O., Jennifer Hahn-Holbrook, Lindsay Chase-Lansdale, Sharon L. Ramey, Julie Krohn, Maxine Reed-Vance, Tonse N. K. Raju, et al. "Racial and Ethnic Differences in Breastfeeding." *Pediatrics* 138, no. 2 (August 2016): e20152388.

Odom, Erika C., Ruowei Li, Kelley S. Scanlon, Cria G. Perrine, and Laurence Grummer-Strawn. "Reasons for Earlier Than Desired Cessation of Breastfeeding." *Pediatrics* 131, no. 3 (March 1, 2013): e726–732.

Paxton Federico, Joanna. "Since the Time of Eve: La Leche League and Communities of Mothers Throughout History." PhD diss., University of Louisville, December 2017.

Perrine, Cria G., Katelyn V. Chiang, Erica H. Anstey, Daurice A. Grossniklaus, Ellen O. Boundy, Erin K. Sauber-Schatz, and Jennifer M. Nelson. "Implementation of Hospital Practices Supportive of Breastfeeding in the Context of COVID-19—United States, July 15–August 20, 2020." *Morbidity and Mortality Weekly Report*. November 27, 2020. www.cdc.gov/mmwr/volumes/69/wr/mm6947a3.htm.

Rich, Adrienne. *Of Woman Born: Motherhood as Experience and Institution*. W. W. Norton & Company, 1986.

Roberts, Dorothy. *Killing the Black Body: Race, Reproduction and the Meaning of Liberty.* Pantheon, 1997.

Sun, Feifei. "Behind the Cover: Are You Mom Enough?" *Time*. May 10, 2012. https://time.com/3450144/behind-the-cover-are-you-mom-enough.

Thomas, Kristen. "It's Time to Retire the Phrase 'Breast Is Best' Once and For All." *Today's Parent*. January 10, 2020. www.todaysparent.com/baby/breastfeeding/yes-breast-is-best-but-its-time-to-retire-that-phrase-once-and-for-all.

Wiessinger, Diane, Diane West, and Teresa Pitman. *The Womanly Art of Breastfeeding*. 8th ed. Ballantine, 2010.

Williams, Florence. *Breasts: A Natural and Unnatural History*. W. W. Norton & Company, 2013.

Williams, Janiya Mitnaul. "Why Black Lactation Matters and the Importance of Black Breastfeeding Week with IBCLC, Janiya Mitnaul Williams." Podcast 189. Evidence Based Birth. August 25, 2021.

Winnicott, Donald. *Winnicott On the Child*. Da Capo Press, 2002.

"Woman Charged After Asking Help Line Breast-Feeding Question." Associated Press. January 18, 1992.

Woodstein, B. J. *The Portrayal of Breastfeeding in Literature*. Anthem Press, 2022.

CHAPTER 10. GOOD ENOUGH

Alcorn, K., A. O'Donovan, J. C. Patrick, D. Creedy, and G. J. Devilly. "A Prospective Longitudinal Study of the Prevalence of Post-Traumatic Stress Disorder Resulting from Childbirth Events." *Psychological Medicine* 40, no. 11 (November 2010): 1849–1859.

Friedman, Matthew. "History of PTSD in Veterans: Civil War to DSM-5." National Center for PTSD. US Department of Affairs. www.ptsd.va.gov/understand/what/history_ptsd.asp.

"How Common Is PTSD in Women?" National Center for PTSD. US Department of Veterans Affairs. www.ptsd.va.gov/understand/common/common_women.asp. Accessed October 18, 2022.

Lamott, Anne. *Operating Instructions: A Journal of My Son's First Year.* Anchor, 2005.

Levine, Peter, and Maggie Kline. *Trauma-Proofing Your Kids: A Parents' Guide to Instilling Confidence, Joy, and Resilience.* North Atlantic Books, 2008.

Oates, M. R., J. L. Cox, S. Neema, P. Asten, N. Glangeaud-Freudenthal, B. Figueiredo, L. L. Gorman, et al. "Postnatal Depression Across Countries and Cultures: A Qualitative Study." *British Journal of Psychiatry* 46 (2004): s10–s16.

Paulson, James F., and Sharnail D. Bazemore. "Prenatal and Postpartum Depression in Fathers and Its Association with Maternal Depression: A Meta-Analysis." *Journal of the American Medical Association* 303, no. 19 (May 19, 2010): 1961–1969.

Popova, Maria. "Pioneering Psychoanalyst Donald Winnicott on the Mother's Contribution to Society." *The Marginalian.* May 8, 2016. www.themarginalian.org/2016/05/08/winnicott-mothers-contribution-to-society.

Raphael-Leff, Joan. "Healthy Maternal Ambivalence." *Studies in the Maternal* 2, no. 1 (January 2010). doi: 10.16995/sim.97.

Schwab, W., C. Marth, and A. M. Bergant. "Post-Traumatic Stress Disorder Post Partum." *Geburtshilfe und Frauenheilkunde* 72, no. 1 (January 2012): 56–63.

Segre, Lisa S., and Wendy N. Davis. "Postpartum Depression and Perinatal Mood Disorders in the DSM." Postpartum Support International. June 2013. www.postpartum.net/wp-content/uploads/2014/11/DSM-5-Summary-PSI.pdf.

A Treatment Improvement Protocol: Trauma-Informed Care in Behavioral Health Services. Publication ID SMA-14-4816. Substance Abuse and Mental Health Services Administration, US Department of Health and Human Services, 2014. https://store.samhsa.gov/sites/default/files/d7/priv/sma14-4816.pdf.

Winnicott, D. W. *Home Is Where We Start From: Essays by a Psychoanalyst.* W. W. Norton and Company, 1990.

Winnicott, Donald. *Winnicott on the Child.* Da Capo Press, 2002.

CHAPTER 11. HOME BIRTH

Some reporting in this chapter appeared in my articles "It's a Scary Time to Have a Baby in a Hospital. Home Births Need to Be More Accessible to Pregnant Women," *Insider*, April 22, 2020, www.insider.com/home-births-should-be-more-accessible-during-the-coronavirus-pandemic-2020-4; and "The Childbirth Photos Instagram Didn't Want You to See," *Harper's Bazaar*, May 11, 2018, www.harpersbazaar.com/culture/a20637023/empowered-birth-project-instagram-censored-birth-photos.

Beynon, Constance. "The Normal Second Stage of Labour: A Plea to Reform Its Conduct." *British Journal of Obstetrics and Gynaecology* 64, no. 6 (December 1957): 815–820.

Brecher, Edward M. *The Sex Researchers.* Little, Brown and Company, 1969.

Caldeyro-Barcia, R., G. Giussi, E. Storch, J. J. Poseiro, N. Lafaurie, K. Kettenhuber, and G. Ballejo. "The Bearing-Down Efforts and Their Effects on Fetal Heart Rate, Oxygenation and Acid Base Balance." *Journal of Perinatal Medicine* 9, Suppl. 1 (February 1981): 63–77.

Fahy, Kathleen, Maralyn Fouruer, and Carolyn Hastie. *Birth Territory and Midwifery Guardianship: Theory for Practice, Education and Research.* Elsevier Health Sciences, 2008.

Haskett, Wendy. "Teacher Gives Pregnancy a Breather." *Los Angeles Times.* March 24, 1987. www.latimes.com/archives/la-xpm-1987-03-24-vw-234-story.html.

Lever, Cindy. "We Are Putting Women Through Torture." *Kidspot.* August 16, 2018. www.kidspot.com.au/birth/labour/real-life/we-are-putting-women-through-torture/news-story/6d4607c77a7a85a4980da4081474d294.

Littlejohn, Marianne. "What Is the Fetal Ejection Reflex?" Spiritual Birth. May 9, 2014. www.spiritualbirth.net/what-is-the-fetus-ejection-reflex.

McCutcheon, Susan. *Natural Childbirth the Bradley Way.* Rev. ed. Plume, 1996.

Newton, N., D. Foshee, and M. Newton. "Experimental Inhibition of Labor Through Environmental Disturbance." *Obstetrics and Gynecology* 27, no. 3 (1966): 371–377.

Newton, Niles. "Fetus Ejection Reflex Revisited." *Birth* 14, no. 2 (1987): 106–108.

Odent, Michael. "Champagne and the Fetus Ejection Reflex." *Midwifery Today* 65 (spring 2003): 9.

Osborne, Kathryn. "Pushing Techniques Used by Midwives When Providing Second Stage Labor Care." PhD diss., Marquette University, 2010.

Osborne, Kathryn, and Lisa Hanson. "Labor Down to Bear Down: A Strategy to Translate Second-Stage Labor Evidence to Perinatal Practice." *Journal of Perinatal & Neonatal Nursing* 28, no. 2 (2014): 117–126.

Wilbur, MaryAnn B., Sarah Little, and Linda Szymanski. "Is Homebirth Safe?" *New England Journal of Medicine.* December 2015.

SOME FURTHER READING

Adichie, Chimamanda Ngozi. *We Should All Be Feminists*

Albert, Elisa. *After Birth*

Allen-Campbell, Yvette, and Suzanne Greenidge-Hewitt. *Black, Pregnant and Loving It: The Comprehensive Pregnancy Guide for Today's Woman of Color*

Allers, Kimberly. *The Big Letdown: How Medicine, Big Business, and Feminism Undermine Breastfeeding*

Allers, Kimberly. *The Mocha Manual to a Fabulous Pregnancy*

Askowitz, Andrea. *My Miserable, Lonely Lesbian Pregnancy*

Austin, Nefertiti. *Motherhood So White: A Memoir of Race, Gender, and Parenting in America*

Baker, Heather. *Homebirth on Your Own Terms: A How-To Guide for Birthing Unassisted*

Beatie, Thomas. *Labor of Love: The Story of One Man's Extraordinary Pregnancy*

Biss, Eula. *On Immunity: An Inoculation*

Caro May, Molly. *Body Full of Stars: Female Rage and My Passage into Motherhood*

Cassidy, Tina. *Birth: The Surprising History of How We Are Born*

Cleghorn, Elinor. *Unwell Women: Misdiagnosis and Myth in a Man-Made World*

Connolly, Maureen. *The Essential C-Section Guide: Pain Control, Healing at Home, Getting Your Body Back, and Everything Else You Need to Know about a Cesarean Birth*

Cusk, Rachel. *Coventry: Essays*

Davis, Angela Y. *Women, Culture & Politics*

Davis-Floyd, Robbie, and Christine Barbara Johnson. *Mainstreaming Midwives: The Politics of Change*

Dekker, Rebecca. *Babies Are Not Pizzas: They're Born, Not Delivered*

DeSilva, Jeremy. *A Most Interesting Problem: What Darwin's Descent of Man Got Right and Wrong About Human Evolution*

Douglas, Susan J. *The Mommy Myth: The Idealization of Motherhood and How It Has Undermined All Women*

Dusenbery, Maya. *Doing Harm: The Truth About How Bad Medicine and Lazy Science Leave Women Dismissed, Misdiagnosed, and Sick*

England, Pam. *Birthing from Within: An Extra-Ordinary Guide to Childbirth Preparation*

Fernyhough, Charles. *A Thousand Days of Wonder: A Scientist's Chronicle of His Daughter's Developing Mind*

Ferrante, Elena. *My Brilliant Friend*

Ferrante, Elena. *The Story of a New Name*

Ferrante, Elena. *The Story of the Lost Child*

Ferrante, Elena. *Those Who Leave and Those Who Stay*

Garbes, Angela. *Like a Mother: A Feminist Journey Through the Science and Culture of Pregnancy*

Gaskin, Ina May. *Ina May's Guide to Childbirth*

Gold, Elizabeth Isadora. *The Mommy Group: Freaking Out, Finding Friends, and Surviving the Happiest Time of Our Lives*

Goldberg, Michelle. *The Means of Reproduction: Sex, Power, and the Future of the World*

Grayson, Jennifer. *Unlatched: The Evolution of Breastfeeding and the Making of a Controversy*

Gross, Jessica. *Screaming on the Inside: The Unsustainability of American Motherhood*

Gross, Rachel E. *Vagina Obscura: An Anatomical Voyage*

Gumbs, Alexis Pauline. *Revolutionary Mothering: Love on the Front Lines*

Gunter, Jen. *The Vagina Bible: The Vulva and the Vagina—Separating the Myth from the Medicine*

Harrington, Kimberly. *Amateur Hour: Motherhood in Essays and Swear Words*

Heti, Sheila. *Motherhood*

Hill, Sarah E. *This Is Your Brain on Birth Control: The Surprising Science of Women, Hormones, and the Law of Unintended Consequences*

Hutter Epstein, Randi. *Get Me Out: A History of Childbirth from the Garden of Eden to the Sperm Bank*

Jung, Courtney. *Lactivism: How Feminists and Fundamentalists, Hippies and Yuppies, and Physicians and Politicians Made Breastfeeding Big Business and Bad Policy*

Klaus, Marshall H. *Mothering the Mother: How a Doula Can Help You Have a Shorter, Easier, and Healthier Birth*

Kolker, Claudia. *The Immigrant Advantage: What We Can Learn from Newcomers to America About Health, Happiness, and Hope*

Lamott, Anne. *Operating Instructions: A Journal of My Son's First Year*

Laurence, Leslie, and Beth Weinhouse. *Outrageous Practices: How Gender Bias Threatens Women's Health*

Leibovitch, Lori. *Maybe Baby: 28 Writers Tell the Truth About Skepticism, Infertility, Baby Lust, Childlessness, Ambivalence, and How They Made the Biggest Decision of Their Lives*

Long Chu, Andrea. *Females*

Manne, Kate. *Down Girl: The Logic of Misogyny*

Martin, Wednesday. *Primates of Park Avenue: A Memoir*

McClain, Dani. *We Live for the We: The Political Power of Black Motherhood*

Nelson, Maggie. *The Argonauts*

Odes, Rebecca, and Ceridwen Morris. *From the Hips: A Guide to Pregnancy, Birth, and Becoming a Parent*

Offill, Jenny. *Department of Speculation*

Orenstein, Peggy. *Waiting for Daisy : A Tale of Two Continents, Three Religions, Five Fertility Doctors, an Oscar, an Atomic Bomb, a Romantic Night, and One Woman's Quest to Become a Mother*

Oster, Emily. *Expecting Better: Why the Conventional Pregnancy Wisdom Is Wrong—and What You Really Need to Know*

Pepper, Rachel. *The Ultimate Guide to Pregnancy for Lesbians: How to Stay Sane and Care for Yourself from Pre-conception Through Birth*

Preece, Bronwyn. *In the Spirit of Homebirth: Modern Women, an Ancient Choice*

Reese, Trystan. *How We Do Family: From Adoption to Trans Pregnancy, What We Learned About Love and LGBTQ Parenthood*

Rich, Adrienne. *Of Woman Born: Motherhood as Experience and Institution*

Roberts, Dorothy. *Killing the Black Body: Race, Reproduction, and the Meaning of Liberty*

Romm, Aviva. *Natural Health After Birth: The Complete Guide to Postpartum Wellness*

Seaman, Barbara. *The Doctors' Case Against the Pill*

Sears, William. *The Breastfeeding Book: Everything You Need to Know About Nursing Your Child from Birth Through Weaning*

Selvaratnam, Tanya. *The Big Lie: Motherhood, Feminism, and the Reality of the Biological Clock*

Slater, Lauren. *Love Works Like This: Moving from One Kind of Life to Another*

Smith Brody, Lauren. *The Fifth Trimester: The Working Mom's Guide to Style, Sanity, and Success After Baby*

Smock, Jessica, and Stephanie Sprenger. *Mothering Through Darkness: Women Open Up About the Postpartum Experience*

Solomon, Anna. *Labor Day: True Birth Stories by Today's Best Women Writers*

Stein, Amy. *Heal Pelvic Pain: A Proven Stretching, Strengthening, and Nutrition Program for Relieving Pelvic Pain, Incontinence, and Other Symptoms Without Surgery*

Stein, Elissa, and Susan Kim. *Flow: The Cultural Story of Menstruation*

Steinem, Gloria. *In Praise of Women's Bodies*

Summers, A. K. *Pregnant Butch: Nine Long Months Spent in Drag*

Thomas, Latham. *Mama Glow: A Hip Guide to Your Fabulous Abundant Pregnancy*

Valenti, Jessica. *Why Have Kids?: A New Mom Explores the Truth About Parenting and Happiness*

Washington, Harriet. *Medical Apartheid: The Dark History of Medical Experimentation on Black Americans from Colonial Times to the Present*

Wertz, Richard, and Dorothy Wertz. *Lying-in: A History of Childbirth in America*

Weschler, Toni. *Taking Charge of Your Fertility: The Definitive Guide to Natural Birth Control, Pregnancy Achievement, and Reproductive Health*

Westervelt, Amy. *Forget "Having It All": How America Messed Up Motherhood—and How to Fix It*

Wolf, Naomi. *Misconceptions: Truth, Lies, and the Unexpected Journey to Motherhood*

Yarrow, Leah. *Parents Book of Pregnancy and Birth*

Zucker, Jessica. *I Had a Miscarriage: A Memoir, a Movement*

INDEX

ABOUT THE AUTHOR

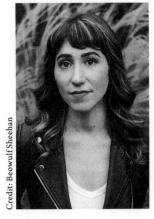

Credit: Beowulf Sheehan

Allison Yarrow is an award-winning journalist, speaker, and author of *90s Bitch*, finalist for the Los Angeles Press Club book award. She was a National Magazine Award finalist, a TED Resident, a producer at NBC News and Vice, a reporter and editor at *Newsweek* and *The Daily Beast*, and her writing and commentary has appeared in many publications. She was raised in Macon, Georgia, and lives with her family in Brooklyn, New York.